DATE DUE

NOV 13			
V 13			

DEMCO 13829810

A Guidebook for
Raising Foster Children

A Guidebook for
Raising Foster Children

Susan McNair Blatt, M.D.
Foreword by Representative Sherwood Boehlert

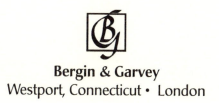

Bergin & Garvey
Westport, Connecticut • London

Library of Congress Cataloging-in-Publication Data

Blatt, Susan McNair, 1945–
 A guidebook for raising foster children / by Susan McNair Blatt ;
foreword by Sherwood Boehlert.
  p. cm.
 Includes bibliographical references and index.
 ISBN 0–89789–653–X (alk. paper)
  1. Foster parents—United States—Handbooks, manuals, etc.
 2. Foster children—Care—United States—Handbooks, manuals, etc.
 3. Foster home care—United States—Handbooks, manuals, etc.
 I. Title.
 HQ759.7.B53 2000
 649'.145—dc21   99–40320

British Library Cataloguing in Publication Data is available.

Library of Congress Catalog Card Number: 99–40320
ISBN: 0–89789–653–X

First published in 2000

Bergin & Garvey, 88 Post Road West, Westport, CT 06881
An imprint of Greenwood Publishing Group, Inc.
www.greenwood.com

Printed in the United States of America

The paper used in this book complies with the
Permanent Paper Standard issued by the National
Information Standards Organization (Z39.48–1984).

10 9 8 7 6 5 4 3 2 1

This book is dedicated to my husband,
Sidney J. Blatt, M.D.

Contents

Contents

Foreword

It would be difficult to think of a more complex, pressing, and emotionally fraught topic than the raising of foster children. Foster children cry out for our attention—our attention as a society as well as our attention as individuals—and to no small extent the future of our society will be influenced by how we respond to that cry.

While we all share the responsibility to respond, it falls most heavily on those dedicated individuals who volunteer to become foster parents. That's why I was so pleased that my friend and neighbor, Dr. Susan Blatt, decided to write this book.

No type of parenting is easy—just go to your local bookstore and you will find shelves groaning with the proliferating advice books on how to raise a child. But although foster parents have more challenges than most—they must deal with a child's often troubling and sometimes only dimly understood past and his or her sense of dislocation—there seem to be far fewer guides out there to help. Foster children sometimes seem to be invisible to society as a whole, despite the crying need to help them and their foster parents.

Yet, foster children are a significant population. According to the U.S. Department of Health and Human Services, there were more than 520,000 children in foster care nationwide—about half of those with non-relatives—at the end of March 1998. With that many children in foster care at any one time, the number of children who have passed through the various state foster care systems is enormous.

Of those 520,000 children, about a quarter were one to five years old, another quarter were between six and ten, and another between 11 and 15. About two-thirds of the children had been in foster care for more than a year, and almost one in five had been in foster care for five years or more. In almost half the cases, the eventual goal was to reunify the child with his or her parents (or other original caretaker).

Foster care is, ideally, a partnership between the government, foster parents, and, in some cases, the birth parents, so looking at government spending is another way to gauge the extent of the foster care system. In fiscal year 1998 (October 1997 through September 1998), total government spending on foster care an estimated $7 billion, according to the U.S. Department of Health and Human Services. Of that $7 billion, about $3.7 billion was spent by the federal government, with the rest coming from states and localities. Spending has been growing; just two years earlier in fiscal 1996, total foster care spending was an estimated $5.6 billion. In recent years, the federal government has expanded the range of its foster care efforts, focusing, in particular, on programs to help older foster care children make the transition to independent living.

Government at all levels is active in foster care for two reasons—one altruistic, the other more pragmatic—both rather self-evident. The altruistic reason is society's humanitarian concern (and I would say obligation) to care for its most vulnerable members. Vice President Hubert Humphrey used to talk about the need to care for those at the dawn of life, at the sunset of life, and in the shadows of life, and it is fitting that the basic federal laws concerning foster care are part of the Social Security Act. The attitudes that spawned the "Great Society" programs of the mid-1960s may now seem quaint, but our societal commitment to foster children and the elderly has not diminished.

The more pragmatic reason is that children who lack a proper and loving upbringing are more likely to impose costs on society later—either by committing crimes, by endangering their own health, or simply by not being fully productive citizens. Nowadays, we often refer to foster children as being "at risk"—and the notion is that they pose a risk to all of us, as well as to themselves.

We need to be careful with such terminology, however, so as not to stigmatize children or care for them in ways that are inappropriate. The history of social welfare policy in this country is in many ways a cautionary tale, as children in the past were too often viewed as requiring outside intervention simply because of their social class, ethnic background, or race.

That history should evoke in all of us a sense of humility, not superiority, as we consider how our predecessors floundered, as we sometimes do, in trying to find the appropriate way to care for children whose parents could not, would not, or did not seem able to do the job. The creation of public schools in the early 19th century, the requirements for compulsory education in the latter part of that century, the creation of work houses and then orphanages (whose residents often had at least one living parent) and even "orphan trains," which resettled Eastern city kids with farm families on the

Great Plains—all of these were efforts to supplement, or substitute, for in-adequacies—real and perceived—in the parenting of at-risk kids.

Foster care is simply the latest, and hopefully best designed, effort of government and non-profit social service agencies to care for our most vulnerable children. By placing children in a family setting, foster care hopes to avoid the failings of institutional care and to give children more sustained, loving, personal attention in an era when it is arguably easier than ever to get lured away from a healthy, productive life.

All this focus on statistics and programs and the risks faced (and posed) by foster children can obscure the very human face of foster care. As foster parents well know, we are talking about real children, each with his or her own strengths and weaknesses, each with the quirks and structures and idiosyncrasies of his or her own personality.

When we talk about foster children as a group, that precious individuality is lost, and we tend to focus unduly on the negative.

One thing I like about Susan's book is that it is alive to the individual nature and variety of foster care and foster children. And that is consistent with my own personal experience. I think my personal story emphasizes two critical points—first, that foster care is not some strange, exotic system, but an extension of informal arrangements that have long existed; and second and more importantly, that children are resilient, that being dubbed "at risk" hardly guarantees any particular outcome.

While I was not formally in any foster care system, I was the child of a young mother who had little notion of how to raise a child. My parents (Dad was a milkman, Mom worked in a meat packing house) were divorced and much of my upbringing was at the hands of my grandmother, who was so strict that she once packed my bags when I refused to eat what she had prepared for dinner. I spent many afternoons alone at the public library; today I guess I would be called a "latchkey" kid, as well.

And yet, despite a difficult childhood and some wasted time in my early 20s, I eventually figured out that I wanted to get serious and went to Utica College in my hometown in upstate New York. From there, I went to Michigan to work for a chemical company and then to Washington as an aide to my local Congressman, beginning a long career of public service. I don't want to hold myself up as any particular type of model, but it's clear that many a child can rise above the circumstances of his or her childhood.

There's no question that excellent foster care can help ensure a happy outcome. I have seen the good done by foster parents in my home area, and their stories are more important than all the statistics in the world. These parents have taken in kids—including kids who had suffered terrible physical or sexual abuse—and within months the children were engaging in new activities, making friends, exploring broader horizons, beginning to put their pasts behind them. Will they still face hurdles in future years? Of course. Will the scars from their past magically vanish? Absolutely not. But they are able to build new, happy lives with the dedicated help and love of their foster parents.

Helen Keller was once asked what things she most regretted not having been able to see. She said, "a child's smile and a sunset."

She was right, of course—there are few things more precious, stunning, and cheering than a child's smile. Foster parents can bring smiles to the faces of children who would otherwise be lost. It is an arduous task; books like this one can help, government programs can help. But in the end, it is the foster parents who do the hard work and share the joy of bringing a smile to a child's face.

Representative Sherwood Boehlert
House of Representatives
Washington, D.C.

Acknowledgments

Many people have offered inspiration and information during this project and it is a pleasure to thank them.

This book is based on discussions with many foster parents, foster children, and former foster children. My favorite interviews were with foster parents who told stories. Their stories are interwoven throughout the book and help to bring the material to life. These folks often had thoughts and suggestions that they wanted to offer to the reader. Their voices are heard, especially, in the last two chapters.

Dr. Joanne Joseph, author of the *Resilient Child*, was extremely helpful in both the subject matter and the writing process. Professionals at the House of the Good Shepherd in Utica, New York, especially William Holicky, executive director, were always thoughtful and helpful.

Susan Cooper, child-life specialist and friend, read much of the book and was quite helpful with content and technicalities. Sylvia Armstrong also read parts of the book and was a source of help and inspiration.

Dr. Thomas Scott got me off to a good start with an understanding of basic psychology of troubled children. Thomas Cutler of the Oneida County Department of Social Services offered a government perspective to the problems of foster care.

My husband, Sidney J. Blatt, MD, was tremendously supportive and encouraging. My daughter, Deborah Blatt, read much of the material with an editor's eye. She also provided the foster puppy, Ned, in our life. Ned is now functioning in the world as a guide dog. My son, Joseph Blatt, reviewed and rewrote the last chapter, advising foster children directly.

My cousin, Patricia Swanson, provided a world of support and encouragement. My mother, Kathryn McNair, who is no longer with us, was an author. Along with my father, J. Dunlap McNair, she encouraged my interest in writing. Good parents themselves, they encouraged me to continue to seek challenges.

The people at the Greenwood Publishing Group, especially Nita Romer, were always there for me when I needed them.

Introduction

If I were a foster parent, I would want a book of directions. Writing such a book turned out to be more difficult than I had expected. I expected to discover published material on this subject as well as research studies that would be helpful. It turned out that published material for those interested in foster care is really not available.

This book of directions is based then, to a large extent, on questions and answers from foster parents. Foster parents have heart-warming stories of their successes and heart-wrenching stories of their frustrations. Listening to foster parents, I was able to focus my research on areas of particular concern.

Foster children also had input into this book. As the pediatrician in a child welfare agency, I have foster children nearby every day. The records of most of these children indicate a troubled past. I listened to these children and learned from them. Their problems are difficult to solve. Former foster children were also ready to talk and to advise. Some are doing well and some are not. I found that a number of former foster children were now foster parents themselves.

The advice and thoughts of foster parents, foster children, and former foster children were integrated with information from professionals. Sometimes I found that the professionals had views quite different from those of the foster parents and foster children. Overall then, the advice in this book is really based on my best judgment.

Many Americans have ideas about the foster care system and how it might be changed for the better. In this book, I chose not to try to change the system. I turned my attention to the day-to-day activities that take place in the half million foster homes in the United States.

Each subject covered in this book begins with a brief description, then considers specific concerns of foster children. There follow concrete suggestions on what you, as a foster parent, can actually do. I know that professional help is not always available for foster parents and I have offered possible approaches to problems, indicating also when a professional should be involved.

Although a foster parent might consider reading straight through the book, most readers will choose to read the appropriate areas. I recommend keeping the book in a convenient location and referring to it for information as situations arise. Very often foster parents will find, upon looking something up, that they have already made good decisions about what to do. In that case, the book can be a comfort.

In the course of writing the book, I gained enormous respect for foster parents. These are people who are willing to "roll up their sleeves and get to work" to help individual foster children. The foster parent who offers a loving home to these children, providing the structure and guidance that the children have missed, will see many small successes with the children. All of us can see the enormous impact that these dedicated adults have on the unfortunate children that spend time in the foster care system.

A Guidebook for
Raising Foster Children

1

Introduction to Foster Care

Whether you are a new foster parent or an experienced foster parent, you will benefit from learning about foster care. Not only will you be prepared for questions from family and friends, but also you will be better able to help your foster child understand what is happening.

Foster care provides substitute homes for children who have been removed from their own homes. Most foster children have been through difficult times and they need care and nurturing by a family that has had special training. There are now approximately 500,000 children in foster care in the United States.

In the past, children without parents were placed in orphanages. It is now considered more appropriate to place such children in private homes. Many children in foster care have parents, but they have been temporarily taken away from those parents. In most cases, the goal for a foster child is reunification with the original family. Various problems that were present at the time the child was removed are addressed while the child is in care.

For some children who enter foster care it becomes apparent that they cannot return to their own biological families, so these children may be offered for adoption. There is a general feeling that this process moves too slowly and laws are in place to try to speed up adoption, moving a child into a permanent home as soon as possible.

WHY CHILDREN BECOME FOSTER CHILDREN

Today about half of all children who are removed from their homes have been abused or neglected. Physical "battering" is the most obvious form of abuse. Neglect is the term for parents not supplying food, clothing, or other needs for the child. Sexual abuse is fairly common. All of these forms of abuse generally are determined as the result of an investigation. If the child's home is found to be unsafe, the child is removed and placed in foster care.

Other children are in foster care because they are considered unmanageable. Such a child may skip school or may roam the streets and get into trouble. The family court judge or juvenile court judge removes the child from the parents. These unmanageable children make up about one quarter of the children in foster care.

A third group of children consists of those who have been abandoned or whose parents cannot care for them. Included in this group are children whose parents are incarcerated or ill. Newborn infants are sometimes abandoned and this may occur as a result of the mother using illegal drugs.

WHAT HAPPENS WHILE A CHILD IS IN FOSTER CARE

In order for the child to return home, the judge usually expects certain improvements in the child's home environment. Birth parents may need to obtain counseling, attend courses, or get jobs. The home situation will be monitored by a social worker or by a probation officer. Based on recommendations from these professionals, the court will decide when a child may return to his or her biological family.

The foster child may also need to change during the period of placement. Foster parents should concentrate on what makes the child likeable and on any strengths the child may have. These traits should be encouraged while negative features of the child's behavior or personality should be discouraged. The child will grow taller, older, and more mature during placement. The encouragement that comes from one's parents or foster parents is a very important part of growing up.

In some situations, the family seems too troubled to take the child back. The parents may offer the child for adoption voluntarily or the child may be freed for adoption as the result of a court decision. This is called "termination of parental rights."

Whether the child eventually returns home or not, foster care represents an opportunity for the child to see how other families live and to know that the future has many options. Foster children often make friends, learn new skills, and develop improved behavior during the time away from their parents.

CHARACTERISTICS OF FOSTER CHILDREN

There are over 500,000 children in out-of-home placement. About 50 percent of these children are Caucasian, 30 percent are African American, and 14 percent are Latino. About 30 percent of foster children are in kinship care, or placement with a relative; that type of foster care is particularly common with African-American families.

About 15 percent of foster children enter care as newborns. Other children are removed from their homes at all ages. About one-third of foster children are removed between birth and age five, one-third between six and twelve, and one-third as teenagers.

Of children who are placed in foster care, 75 percent are in regular foster homes, 15 percent are in group homes or institutions, and the rest are in various other settings. Runaway youth, children living with neighbors or friends, children in homeless shelters, and children living independently are not in foster care and are not considered "placed." These youngsters may represent an additional half million children.

The average length of stay in foster care is one and a half years. However, some children may stay in foster care for many years. Two-thirds of children who leave foster care are reunited with their own families. Adoption occurs in about 10 percent of cases. Fifteen percent of children entering care have been in foster care in the past. Some children leave the foster care system to become independent, usually at age eighteen.

CHARACTERISTICS OF BIOLOGICAL FAMILIES

When a child is removed from the biological parents, a judge has decided that the environment is harmful for the child. Generally such families are quite poor and often there is no father in the home. Alcohol, drugs, crime, violence, and jail are common themes with such families.

Birth parents of foster children often admit that they are poor disciplinarians. "I just didn't know how to make my kids behave," said one such mother. They ignore good behavior and overreact to bad behavior. They shout and hit when they feel that the child is misbehaving. Such an upbringing often results in children who are disruptive and difficult to manage.

Frequently, birth mothers were teenagers when they had their first child. They tried to raise that child and soon had another. Lack of adult guidance, lack of money, and lack of parenting skills resulted in troubled homes for such young families.

Unmarried women raising young children may allow men to move into the home. In such homes, there is often abuse of children and violence toward adult women. Weapons may be readily available. "When I visited the birth home, mom's boyfriend was there and he had a knife sticking out of his back pocket," said one caseworker.

These biological parents almost always indicate that they love their children and wish they could offer them more advantages. A young mother, overwhelmed by poverty and fearing the violence around her, may accept the temporary removal of her children. Such a mother may enter a drug rehabilitation program, get a job, or move the boyfriend out of the home, and then the children can return to a more stable environment.

EXPECTATIONS FOR THE BIRTH FAMILY DURING FOSTER CARE

Resources for troubled families tend to be focused on foster children, rather than on the biological family of that child. Although agencies have a history of providing a complete program of services for foster children, the child's biological family generally is not offered a span of services. Such a family with poverty, lack of education, illegal drug use, and domestic violence is often expected to "pull itself together."

It is expected that more services will be available to these troubled families in the near future. Government leaders have realized that these particular families can benefit from the same attention as their children. Programs designed to keep children out of foster care and "family-strengthening" programs are available in some communities. As agencies develop skills to work with such families, there should be improvement in the future.

In the meantime, agencies do try to help troubled families put together a program that is acceptable. There are usually court-ordered requirements for the parents, such as drug rehabilitation programs, which must be met before the child can return. Families may be required to participate in programs, or may voluntarily find programs, to help them become better parents. A birth parent may take this time to learn to read, to get a high school diploma, or to gain job skills.

While a child is in foster care, the biological family may learn about programs that are available and expert help for them to turn to in the future. The biological parents may have learned how to use their own extended family for help, especially if they have participated in kinship foster care. It is also quite common for a biological parent to stay in communication with former foster families and turn to a former foster parent for guidance or advice.

DIFFICULT BEHAVIOR OF FOSTER CHILDREN

It can be assumed that children who are taken away from their homes have had a difficult time. Many such children have been neglected or abandoned, and others have been abused. Almost all have lacked the consistent, nurturing care that most Americans provide for their children. It is hard to comprehend fully the impact of years of mistreatment.

Certain characteristics are common in children who have been through bad experiences. Many foster children act older than might be expected. Often they have had to take care of themselves, and such a child may have been the most "grown-up" person in the household. Such a child may seem stubborn and opinionated and may not be willing to listen to foster parents. On the other hand, foster children may sometimes seem immature. Problems like bed-wetting and temper tantrums are quite common. Often the child has simply not been in a stable environment at the time that these behaviors should have ended.

Foster children often are not committed to telling the truth. They may tell lies in harmful ways or they may tell casual untruths. They may have lied so much in the past that they are not sure what is the truth. Sometimes they may make up elaborate stories that represent the way they wish things were.

Most disturbing is the anger that many foster children have and the ways they may express this anger. Anger may be aimed at siblings, pets, teachers, or foster parents. An angry foster child may become aggressive. Foster children may think that it is all right for them to hit someone, because they have been hit in the past.

It is challenging to raise someone else's child, especially when that child has gotten off to a difficult start. Helping a child who has been treated badly in the past is difficult but extremely rewarding. One foster parent said, "I would do anything for that kid, to make sure that life treats him fairly, from now on."

Although foster children may be difficult to raise, they also have good features. A foster child may make you proud and will often make you smile or laugh. As a foster parent, you will be deeply satisfied as you help the child learn new behaviors that will make him or her stronger. Your goal is to take a child into your home and help that child develop increased resiliency, to make him or her strong and able to bounce back.

ORPHANAGES

Many years ago, society had little sympathy for children without parents. These children might have been put into orphanages or into private homes. They needed to work in the institution or in the home to "earn their keep." Gradually, the system changed so that foster parents were paid the child's expenses and the child was not expected to work for the family. During the depression, in the 1930s, the federal government took on some of the financial responsibility for these children.

At the present time, foster children are in the custody of their county and state. Guardianship usually remains with the biological parents. The federal government continues to cover much of the cost. Instead of government departments, child welfare agencies may accept the care of foster children. Foster families are paid the child's expenses. In special situations, the foster family may receive additional money.

One reason that foster care took the place of orphanages is that children who grew up in orphanages became "institutionalized." These children did not learn how to be part of a family. One woman said, "My husband was raised in an orphanage and he had a terrible time raising kids. Everything seemed new to him. Now he's doing better, as a grandfather."

An orphanage was considered a permanent placement. Such facilities no longer exist, and most childcare experts agree that orphanages should not exist. It is felt that foster children should be placed in the most homelike setting in which they can be safe and happy. This is called the least restrictive environment. The foster home should be as similar as possible to the child's birth home.

INSTITUTIONS FOR CHILDREN

There are still institutions for children, but almost always placement in these facilities is considered temporary. One type of facility is called a residential treatment center. These usually have fifty to two hundred children, who live and go to school there. The children are too disturbed or too disturbing to manage in foster care. Residential treatment centers are part of the child welfare system.

Most communities have group homes, run by child welfare agencies. These are often located in residential neighborhoods amid other private homes. The children may stay there for several years and they generally go to public school. There are various specialized group homes, such as those for pregnant teenaged girls.

Children in the juvenile justice system may be placed in detention. These facilities vary from state to state. Youngsters in such facilities should not be in communication with adults who are incarcerated. At the present time, there are about 100,000 children in detention in the United States.

Children who are mentally retarded are generally not institutionalized. Either they remain in their own homes or they may be placed in substitute homes. Mentally disturbed or mentally ill children are generally handled in the child welfare system unless there is a need for psychiatric hospitalization. After such hospitalization, if their conditions improve, they may be discharged back to their homes or into foster homes.

In all such facilities there is oversight to prevent neglect or abuse. The government agency that funds these facilities maintains supervision over food, clothing, and other necessities. Counseling and other help for improving behavior is usually provided. These institutions are not entirely homelike. Staff members generally work on a shift system. Meals and activities are not always family-style. So for most children in institutions, the goal is to move them into a more homelike setting.

CHARACTERISTICS OF FOSTER PARENTS

Generally, people become foster parents because they feel that they have something to offer to these children. They accept the long hours of responsibility and attention. They receive enough money to take care of the child, but seldom make a profit. Most foster families are two-parent families. They have a home with some extra space. Often their own children are a little older. Interestingly, many foster parents had grown up with foster children in their own homes. Some foster parents are single parents. Usually such a person has some extended family nearby for support. Sometimes older people become foster parents. Kinship foster care involves the placement of a child with relatives.

Many African Americans become foster parents, providing appropriate homes for African-American youngsters. Agencies try to place children in environments where they will be most comfortable. Persons who are bilingual provide a very special advantage for a bilingual child as communication can be maintained with the biological family.

Foster parents with special skills, such as nursing, may be able to care for certain chronically ill children who would otherwise not be able to be placed in a home situation. Foster families may receive additional funding for such a child. Teachers, clergy, social workers, and others in "helping professions" are very likely to become foster parents.

New foster parents take a course that meets regularly for several weeks. They discuss all aspects of child care with other prospective foster parents and with professionals. Each foster parent has a physical exam, certain routine health screening tests are done, and the home is inspected. On successful completion of these tests, they are licensed to be foster parents.

WHETHER OR NOT TO BECOME FOSTER PARENTS

Most families go into foster care because they genuinely want to work with other families and help "put them back together." Very few families go into foster care as a way to make money. As a prospective foster parent, you need to be sure that your motivation is reunification of troubled families. You need a safe and roomy house, acceptable transportation, and good health. Foster parents who work outside the home will need extra energy at the end of the workday to deal with a foster child.

Taking in foster children may seem like a big step at the beginning, and it is often hard to predict whether it is something you and your family can do successfully. You need to talk to everyone who lives in the household to make sure that they can make the commitment of time, energy, and love. Think about how you and your spouse handled difficult times in the past. If your own children were sometimes more than you could handle, think twice about foster parenting. However, if you have successfully raised your own children and most of the time things went smoothly, then move ahead with your plan.

The most important thing foster parents do is give their time and their attention. Can you listen to a child consistently? Can you advise a child in a practical way? Can you be available when he or she wants to talk, wants to work things out, or wants to dream about the future? Can you be a loving substitute parent, even when a child is being difficult?

Many Americans want to adopt a child. Most foster parents would recommend not getting into foster care if you really want to adopt. Children rarely become adoptable and, when they do, their own relatives usually have the right to adopt them.

DIFFERENT TYPES OF FOSTER CARE

Each state or area has its own names for types of foster care. Regular foster care is often called "family foster care," a term used to distinguish it from institutional care. In most areas, a single training course with about eight sessions is a necessary requirement for foster parents, with a few updates every year thereafter. "Kinship foster care" is similar to regular foster care except that the foster parent is a relative of the child. Informal kinship care not arranged through an appropriate agency is not foster care and no special payment is made to the caregivers.

A more intense level of foster care may be called specialized foster care, therapeutic foster care, or treatment foster care. In this situation, the child is more troubled and the foster parents receive more training. Foster parents participate actively in the management of the child in this level of care. They work together with the therapeutic team to devise treatment plans. This form of foster care is more expensive and these foster parents are paid more.

A new form of foster care is called "shared family foster care." In this case, the entire biological family, often a single-parent family, moves into the foster home. This may be done with young mothers, mothers with low intelligence, or mothers who have used drugs. In this type of care the child is able to stay with his or her parents and the outcomes may be quite good.

There are other types of special foster care for several specific types of children, such as those who are mentally retarded, mentally disturbed, or juvenile delinquents. Different agencies handle different types of these placements, and each agency has its own specific requirements.

METHODS FOR STRENGTHENING BIRTH FAMILIES

For most foster placements, the goal is to return the child to his or her original home. Does this make sense? Of course you love your own children and you want them to stay with you. If you look at the foster child's biological family that way, you realize that home is usually the best place for a child. Biological parents who show signs of improving their lifestyle, as required by the judge, deserve a second chance.

The social worker, caseworker, or probation officer is involved in helping people to improve various skills. That is done in three ways: by teaching, by modeling, and by setting reasonable goals.

Parents whose children have been taken away are able to attend parenting classes offered in various agencies. Studies indicate that adults can be taught new ways of raising children and of managing their own lives. Modeling is provided in the foster home where the child is able to see appropriate family interactions. Unfortunately, caseworkers often fail to bring the biological family to the foster home. If the two families are brought together, the birth family may show significant improvement, just by watching the foster family interact. Goals for the family are usually set by the judge and may include family visitations, drug rehabilitation, getting a job, or moving to a safer home. Each of these requirements, when met, moves the family nearer to reunification.

METHODS FOR HELPING FOSTER CHILDREN CHANGE

A child in foster care has an opportunity to learn new behaviors and new attitudes. He or she is growing up while in the foster home. Foster families can influence youngsters to help them behave better and become more responsible. The same three techniques, teaching, modeling, and goal setting, are used for improving the child's behavior.

First, the child is taught about family life. The foster parent explains how the foster child should act and why the child should follow rules and behave well. When problems occur, such as an argument between two children, foster parents teach a better way to get along. Second, foster families provide a model of a normal family for the child. The child sees how your family gets along and learns from it. Third, goals are set for the child. The professionals may help with this, and foster parents may be involved in encouraging the child to meet the goals that have been set.

Ideally, as the biological family begins to deal with the problems and stresses of their lives, the home becomes a more suitable place for the foster child. At the same time, the foster child has had an opportunity to grow and change and learn new behaviors so that there will be success when the family reunites.

FOSTER CHILDREN LEARN ABOUT FAMILIES

Foster children need to know the pleasures and challenges of family life. Your family may have its good days and its bad days. The important thing is that the foster child should see how the entire family deals with issues and stresses. It is especially important when family members disagree among themselves that someone explains to the foster child what is happening. This allows the child to understand how differences are worked out in healthy families.

Many foster children have not been exposed to activities that your children take for granted. A trip in the car, dinner in a restaurant, or a game of tennis may be a new experience for this child. Try to explain these activities and help the child by planning ahead. School will present challenges for the child and you should indicate that you will help with school problems as best you can. The ways you have handled your own children and their school problems will help you with a foster child.

Whatever your family's religion, talk to the child and caseworker about the child's participation. You may need to arrange for the child's involvement in a religion that is not your own. Other cultural, ethnic, and racial issues may have to be addressed as well. The child may feel that your family members are involved in activities very different from those he or she grew up with. At the same time, this child's heritage may be foreign to your family. Try to learn as much as you can about the child's culture and encourage expression of that culture in your home. Plan carefully for major holidays and work with the caseworker to make sure that the biological parents are also involved. Holiday times can be quite troublesome for foster children and for their families.

A foster home does not need to be a perfect home. It should, however, be a home with love and strong bonds. There should be a willingness to sit down and talk over problems that arise.

TERMINATION OF PARENTAL RIGHTS

Parents may give up their children for adoption when they feel they cannot raise them. This can occur with newborns or with older children. Sometimes parents are doing children a huge favor by allowing adoption to proceed. The caseworker and judge will make the arrangements for termination of parental rights.

Sometimes birth parents try to meet the various requirements set forth by the judge, but they do not succeed. If the court's requirements are not met, the court will terminate the birth parents' rights. Sometimes there are long delays in this complicated process. The biological parents may cause the delays if they do not want to give up the child. An additional delay usually occurs between termination and adoption. This period averages two to three years in most localities. There is a strong feeling among many professionals and foster parents that this process does not happen fast enough.

At the same time, most Americans agree that children should not be completely cut off from parental involvement. Studies show that it is generally beneficial for a child to maintain ties with his or her biological parents even if parental rights have been terminated. In actual experience, many families do maintain such a relationship. One former foster mother said,

"Carrie's birth mother calls me about once a month and so does her adoptive mother. I keep communication open between the two moms. Right now Carrie does not really want to see her birth mom, but when she does, I'll help make the arrangements."

There are many concerns around the issue of termination of parental rights, and it seems unlikely that there will be dramatic changes soon. The time a child spends in your home should not be just a waiting period before adoption. It should be a time of change and growth for that child, so that whether or not adoption occurs, the child will be stronger.

ADOPTING FOSTER CHILDREN

There are several ways that foster children may end up being adopted. Sometimes, if the biological parent has voluntarily given up the child, the child will be placed in foster care temporarily while the paperwork and waiting periods are completed. In other situations, the birth parents do not meet goals set by the judge and court proceedings are begun to terminate parental rights involuntarily. A third situation concerns abandoned children, who are usually placed in foster care for a certain period before adoption.

In all of these situations, the court will give preference to family members of the child. In other words, even if the child has been in your home for many months, when he or she is freed for adoption, the judge may place the child with an aunt or grandmother. Also, brothers and sisters who have been placed in different foster homes may be brought together into one adoptive home in order to keep the siblings together.

Any time you are considering adoption, you should find out as much as possible about the background of the child. Ask the doctor about any health problems. Ask the caseworker if, after adoption, you will receive financial assistance for the child. With most hard-to-place children there is federal funding to subsidize adoption. This subsidy will continue throughout the childhood of the youngster you adopt.

Start discussing your plan to adopt with your spouse. You and your spouse need to be in agreement. Your relatives may also express opinions, as will your own children. You will want to keep these discussions confidential. Do not allow the child to think you are going to adopt him or her until you are sure.

REMOVAL OF FOSTER CHILDREN FROM FOSTER HOMES

A foster child may leave your home for several reasons. The child may be returned to the biological family, may run away or drift away, or may be moved to a different foster home or to an institution.

A child goes home to his or her biological family when the judge determines that the child will be safe and comfortable there. Usually the caseworker has a lot of influence on this decision and if you are communicating well with the caseworker, you will be well informed. Children sometimes know that they have a court date. If it appears that the child may be sent home, try to work with the child so that the transition back home will be smooth.

In some situations, the judge may move the child to another foster home. There are several reasons for this type of move. A child might be moved to be with siblings, with relatives, or near the biological family. On the other hand, siblings sometimes cannot seem to live together in one foster home. If this happens, it may become necessary to separate them.

Another possibility is that the placement is not working out well and the foster family has asked that the child be sent to another foster home or has recommended placement in an institution. Once in a while, children ask to leave a particular foster home. They may feel they are being mismanaged or even abused. When an allegation of abuse is made to the authorities, the child is usually moved to another home.

Sometimes foster parents are warned about impending moves. There may be time to talk things through with the child, arrange future communication, and have a going-away party. In other cases, the judge may make a sudden decision and the foster parents are taken by surprise. Try to anticipate all the options and help the child deal with the outcome. Every effort should be made to help the child feel comfortable with the caseworker, because that person will lead the child through the entire placement experience.

FEELINGS WHEN A FOSTER CHILD LEAVES

People who are unfamiliar with foster care often ask if it will be difficult to give up the child. There is no easy answer to the question. Most foster children stay in their first placement less than a year and remain in foster care less than two years. Consequently, there is a lot of movement of foster children.

In some cases it is fairly easy to accept a child leaving. The child may go back to a home that has improved, go to live with a grandmother, or may be adopted. In these situations, foster parents are usually contented to watch the child move out; often they will arrange to maintain contact in the future. In other cases, the child seems to be moving back to an unsafe home, or he or she is being moved to another foster home and the reason is not clear to the foster family. This type of move is unsettling. However, there is a lot of coming and going in a busy foster home, and foster parents usually get used to it.

The second question people ask is, Will we get too attached? Again, this is usually not an issue for foster parents who have been in the business for

many years. One foster mother said, "My goal was to give them as much as I could before they went back. I've had about sixteen of them and I know where most of them are. They're doing all right." If you are new to foster care and you are concerned about becoming too attached, review your motivations for becoming a foster parent. If your motivation is to help troubled families get back together, then attachment will be less of a concern.

Some foster children maintain ties with their former foster parents. "Eric had lived with us for three years when he was sent to live with an aunt. He and his cousin visited me every few weeks until they were grown up. I went with him to rent his first tux. I'm still holding onto a savings account we started, because he wants me to," said a former foster father.

Do not expect words of appreciation from the child. These children have been through some hard times, and they seldom express their appreciation in ways you might desire. However, if they have had some success at school, or made a friend, or learned a new skill, it is because of the good care you provided.

After you have taken a number of foster children into your home, you will get used to them coming and going. Still, you will remember each child and the love you offered that child during the time of placement in your home.

2

Welcoming
New Foster Children

Usually there is little opportunity to prepare for a foster child before the child arrives at your home. The caseworker drops off the child with his or her records and possessions. Foster parents and foster children agree that it is important to get off to the right start.

Try to allow some extra time the first few days and weeks for gathering together information on the child, for helping him or her get adjusted to the family and school, and just for sitting and talking. Your attention and interest in the first few weeks will set a pattern. The child will know that you care about him or her and that you are willing to help with any issues that he or she wishes to share with you.

INFORMATION ABOUT THE CHILD

When a new foster child is brought to your home, you will be given a packet of materials. You need information about the child, about the child's schooling, and about the child's health. You need the social security number, birth certificate, and data about the birth parents. Ask for the child's full name, nicknames, and any other last names that the child might have used. Sometimes part of this material is missing. The caseworker should bring the rest to you when it becomes available.

Certain information is helpful in starting a child in a new school. You should have the name of the old school, the grade level, and the type of classroom. Sometimes the child will be able to help with this. Medical records are also important. You must know details of any medication that is being used and of any allergies. Immunization records should come with the child. It is helpful to have the name of the doctor or clinic. It is important to understand chronic health problems such as asthma and ear infections.

Lastly, find out as much as you can about the child's interests. Pay close attention to any information about the child's strengths. What skills does he or she have? Does he or she have any particular fears? Are there behavior problems you should know about immediately?

Take a large envelope and write the child's name on it. As you gather information about the child, keep a copy of each item in the folder. Add items such as photographs and school papers as time goes by. This folder can then stay with the child when he or she leaves your home.

WHAT TO DO IN THE FIRST FEW HOURS

After the caseworker leaves, it is time to sit down and talk with the child. Try to remove all other family members except your spouse. Ask the child questions and wait patiently for the answers. Certain questions will immediately make the child feel better, and others might cause discomfort. Try to avoid uncomfortable questions.

Former foster children often talk about this first moment with a new foster parent as a very important time. The following are suggestions from former foster children. Do not indicate that your rules will be rigid. Do not discuss chores. Do not indicate that the foster child will be treated differently from the biological children in the home. Know that children worry about their own safety. The child may be worried that you will neglect her, treat her badly, or abuse her. Be reassuring about that.

After your initial talk, show the child around the house, introducing the other children, the adults, and the pets. Suggest a snack that will feel like a treat to the child. Food is a very important part of all relationships. Sitting down with a new child and having a snack with her is a wonderful way to begin.

In the first evening, talk to the child about bedtime. See what time she normally goes to bed and whether or not she sleeps with a light on. Make sure she can get to the bathroom at night and knows how to call you. Expect her to be a little scared at bedtime when the house is dark and quiet. Check on her and, if necessary, sit with her until she goes to sleep.

In all likelihood, you and your spouse are a little nervous about welcoming a new child to your home. You are concerned about whether or not you will all get along and whether you can keep the child safe. The child will have similar concerns and, indeed, the child may be quite frightened. Strive to be pleasant and welcoming on this important first day.

GETTING STARTED WITH SCHOOL

If school is in session, the child needs to be taken to school very shortly after arrival. Many children feel more settled once they have started school.

If this child has not already changed schools often, talk with her about going to a new school. Mention that the work may seem hard at first, as everything will be new.

When you take the child to school, be sure to meet the teacher. Say very positive things about the child. Tell the teacher what a great child this is and mention some way that she has pleased you. Do this in front of the child. It is acceptable to exaggerate a little when you are praising a child. Ask the teacher to call you soon and let you know how the child is doing. If the child has severe behavior problems, mention that to the teacher in private. If there are illnesses or medications, talk to the school nurse.

Talk to the child about getting to know the children in the new school. If possible, find a neighborhood child who will be in her class to befriend your foster child. Tell the child that the other children may tease her and that she should try not to let it be upsetting. Tell the child that everyone expects to feel a little scared on the first day in a new school.

TALKING THINGS OVER AT THE BEGINNING

You need to be available to listen and talk with a new foster child. Even though events in the child's life may have been very chaotic, he or she may not have much to say about the past for a while. In the first few days, you should set a pattern of communication that will allow the child to talk to you about more serious things later.

The foster child needs to do a lot of talking and that means you need to do a lot of listening. Allow some quiet time the first few days to learn about this child. Ask the child how the day went and wait patiently for the answer. As the child learns that you are truly interested, he or she will begin to open up. "The first day or two she didn't say anything, and now I can't stop her. She's a regular chatterbox," said one foster mother.

As a foster parent, you need to help this child grow. All children must become stronger and more independent as they get older. It is especially important that this child learns to speak up for herself and to get along in the world, as the child's own parents may not be there for her.

Even at the beginning, there are ways to encourage a child to be strong and self-reliant. Ask about details of the day. If she showed any evidence of strength or wisdom, praise the child for that. "I'm so glad you figured out how to ask for juice instead of milk. You're really getting off to a good start. You need to remember that you are allergic to milk," is an example of such a comment.

HELPING A FEARFUL CHILD

Anxiety and fearfulness are quite common in foster children. This is especially true when a child is in a new foster home. Some fears that foster children have are quite reasonable, such as worrying that they will be lonely. Foster parents help a new foster child by being affectionate, ready to listen, and ready to reassure. Many foster children are fearful that they will be abused. Abuse is a difficult subject to discuss in the first few days of a new placement. Yet, for the child who has been abused, some assurance must be made that he or she will be safe in your home.

Fear of the dark is quite common when children first arrive and it can occur at any age. Talk about the problem during the day and try to work out some solutions for the child. Talk about using a night-light, playing a radio, or leaving a door open.

School is often frightening for foster children. They may worry about academic failure or they may be afraid of the other children. These fears are quite realistic and will generally be overcome after the first few weeks.

Separation is always hard. Foster children have been separated from their birth families, and they may be fearful that they will never live with their original family again. Also, they may fear leaving a foster home and being separated from the foster family. Separation issues are common concerns among foster children.

There is only so much you can do to relieve the anxieties of a new foster child. You cannot promise that you will always take care of her. Tell the child that she will become more comfortable as she stays with you and that you will keep her as safe as you can.

FOSTER FAMILY'S NEED TO ADJUST

If this is your first foster child, the experience may be somewhat stressful for you and your family. A new child will bring a certain amount of noise and confusion. Your old patterns of daily activities may have to change. Your own biological children may be disturbed by the presence of an additional child. Sometimes extended family or neighbors become involved and then criticize you or the foster child. Grandparents may be upset at the thought of having to adjust to another "grandchild."

Taking in a foster child may test the strength of your marriage. Do not be surprised if you find yourselves arguing with each other over problems about the child. With patience, this will usually resolve itself.

A badly behaved foster child may result in phone calls from teachers, comments from neighbors, and a feeling of frustration on your part. The role of the caseworker is to help with the transition of this child into your home. Take advantage of this person or any other professionals who are available to you.

If a new foster child is ill upon arrival or becomes ill in the first few days, there may be the additional confusion of identifying a doctor or clinic for the child. During moments such as this, you may need help from other family members to give you time to resolve the problems confronting you and the child.

MAKING A HOME SAFE FOR FOSTER CHILDREN

Take a survey of your home and see if this child will be safe in it. Be sure to lock up matches, lighters, and weapons. For young children, put safety plugs in sockets and latches on cupboards. Lock up medications and put fragile items out of reach. If the foster child is a baby, make sure your own children and your pets do not harm the child.

If the new child is a toddler, make sure there are no small objects on the floors and move medicines and cleaning supplies up high. Consider protecting the stairs with a gate. Use an approved carseat and make sure it is installed correctly. If you have a swimming pool or a trampoline, make sure the child does not have access to it.

As a foster parent cares for a child, the child is also growing and changing. New safety issues will arise as the child grows older. It is a serious responsibility to keep a child safe.

SPECIAL HOUSEHOLD RULES

A family that is taking in extra children needs to have certain basic rules and these rules need to apply to everyone. You may or may not want to post a list of rules. Former foster children have said that such a list of rules can be unpleasant when presented in the first few hours. Rules should be part of the way your family runs, but they should not require much discussion at the beginning. Foster children can be quite comfortable with rules that the whole family follows. Foster children are uncomfortable with rules that apply only to them or with rules that are not followed.

Your family's special rules may or may not include the following. Notice that these are rules about safety, health, and respect and apply to everyone in the home. Make sure that your spouse and your own children are in agreement and can live with these rules.

- No one hits anyone else
- No one smokes inside the house
- No one runs inside the house
- Children go to school every day unless they are sick
- No child uses matches or lighters unless supervised
- Everyone uses seat belts when in cars
- Always respect others
- Do not steal

BEHAVIOR CONCERNS AT THE BEGINNING

Try to get a quick overview of this child's behavior from the caseworker. Ask about any areas of particular concern, such as aggressiveness or tantrums. Also, try to listen for good aspects of this child's behavior. As your job is to improve the child's behavior, you will be building on the good behavior that he demonstrates. Ask if there are certain activities or suggestions that will help this child behave well.

Some foster children will have developed a reputation for trouble in other foster homes. This behavior may or may not occur while the child is in your care. If the child can learn to listen to you and trust you, the same troubles may never arise in your home. A foster child may act up in order to see how you react. If this happens in the first few days, tell him that the behavior is not acceptable and then try not to show much reaction. "Phil broke a vase on the second day he was with us. I saw him do it and he knew I saw him. I was kind of casual about it. I figured we would talk about it later," said a foster mother.

Find out from the caseworker if the child sees a specialist for behavior or if he is on any behavior medication. If the child is followed by such a specialist, ask when the next appointment is and how to reach that person.

Physical activity is a good antidote for challenging behavior. Take the child out and throw a ball back and forth. When the child comes in and is physically tired, the disruptive behavior may not start again. Quiet conversations with just the two of you will also be helpful. A snack together will allow the child to know that you are his friend and that you are not angry.

FOLLOWING DIRECTIONS

In healthy families, parents and children tend to get along. This may occur because, as babies, they learned that obeying their parents brought praise. Your foster child may not have received that kind of attention from his own parents. From the beginning, when this child is quite new, consider ways to form a good relationship with the child. Try to give suggestions rather than directions. This avoids confrontations when a child does not wish to comply. It allows you the option of "giving in" if the issue does not seem important.

There will, of course, be areas where you will expect obedience. Try to plan ahead with discussions of these areas. If you do not want the child to ride a bike in the street, tell him that. If he rides his bike in the street anyway, say that he will have to stay closer to you for a while so you can keep him safe.

You may have a "honeymoon period" when the child follows your directions; then, at some point, the child may begin to test the strength of your resolve. If the child appears to be testing you, be firm and quiet. Try to make it easy for the child to decide to comply with your wishes. Make sure that the child gets positive reinforcement for following directions. If he does not obey, do not make a fuss. If the child is relatively normal, this approach will result in a healthy relationship between you and the child. If problems persist, you will need to talk to the caseworker.

GETTING STARTED WITH HEALTH CARE

Very soon after arrival, the child should be seen by the doctor. You need to establish a connection in case of ill health. You also need certain kinds of information, such as previous illnesses. Try not to let more than a week or two go by before making an appointment at a clinic or doctor's office.

Many children fear doctors and a new foster child will be naturally uneasy. Younger children may fuss and struggle and older children may be quite unhappy. Talk about the visit ahead with the child. The child may very well need updates on immunizations, so do not say that there will or will not be shots. Just promise that you will be there and that the doctor will understand. Many children entering foster care are behind in their immunizations. This may be because of neglect on the part of parents. However, it also may be because of changing requirements and recommendations.

Most foster children are not enrolled in the kind of health insurance program that your own family is likely to be in. Instead they are in whatever health care system your state has for those on public assistance. The services provided are usually adequate, but often there are limitations as to the doctor or clinic you can use. If the child had a good relationship with a health care provider before coming to you, consider staying there. Otherwise, see if the doctor who takes care of your own children can take this child. Nurse practitioners will often see the child. However, if the child is ill, a doctor or a specialist may be needed. Make sure you know whom to call at night and which emergency room to use, should a problem arise.

If the child is quite ill, you may need to go to an emergency room in the first few days of placement. The child may have been through experiences that make him more fearful than you realize. Try to stay with him as much as possible. The child will be comforted by your presence and you will know what happened during the visit. Try to get medical directions in writing, and be sure to call your caseworker the next day.

When you take the child for the first physical examination, ask that records of height, weight, vision, hearing, tuberculosis test, and immunizations be written down for you to keep. Talk about any health concerns you or the child may have. Add the records you receive at that visit to your child's folder at home.

NUTRITION REVIEW

Take a look at a new foster child. If the child is of normal size and normal weight, he probably knows how much to eat. However, his choice of foods may need improvement. If the child is overweight, he will probably continue to eat too much at your house unless you help. If the child is underweight, there are two possibilities. One is the natural thinness that occurs in some families and is not a sign of ill health. The other is that some children are malnourished because they are neglected. If a child is small and thin and has a history of neglect, he or she may catch up in size while with you.

While you have the child, you will be trying to change many habits and behaviors, including some food-related behaviors. Table manners can be a problem for a child who has been raised in a turbulent home environment. Be firm, but patient regarding use of utensils and portion size. The child may need to grow up a little before cooperating with this.

Many children who have grown up in poverty have not learned to eat fruits and vegetables. Five servings a day is recommended, but if that does not seem possible, work on one or two servings of fruits or vegetables and then increase gradually to five. If the child has food allergies and has had serious allergic reactions in the past, you will have to be very careful. The child also may have strong likes and dislikes regarding foods. It is important to consider any cultural differences in eating habits.

EXPECTATIONS

Foster children need to know what you expect. On the other hand, the children may have their own expectations for their experience, so expectations need to be considered on both sides. Your expectations for the child should be realistic from the beginning. You should expect the basic rules of the household to be followed, and you will have daily expectations about the child getting home at mealtimes and so on. You should expect reasonable cooperation with activities in the home, and an older child should be expected to take care of his or her own room and clothing. You and your family expect to be treated with respect by the foster child.

The foster child expects a private space, food, and clothing. She also expects to be safe from harm. The child expects guidance from you in all aspects of her life. She deserves encouragement when discouraged and respect when troubled.

What foster parents should not expect is a young person to do the chores, a perfectly behaved child, or a child who expresses appreciation to the foster parents on a daily basis. They should not expect any more success in school than the child is capable of. They should not expect the child to join them in their religious activities or to agree with them on every issue.

If you ask a foster child what he or she expects out of life, you may be surprised to hear an elaborate plan. A girl wants to be a beautician and have a shop and a husband and a baby. It is human nature that children have high expectations for their own future. It is important to respect children and encourage them. Show them the steps that will be necessary for fulfilling their future goals and help them on their way.

HELPING A FOSTER CHILD LEARN TO TRUST

Children from normal families learn to trust their parents in the first year and a half of life. The result of developing trust in parents is to begin to develop trust in others. In other words, experience teaches trust. However, the experiences of foster children may have been very hurtful. Their parents may have lied to them, abused them, or abandoned them. Learning to trust others will be a slow process.

Learning trust is a process that involves a series of bargains. With a child in a normal family, the mother puts her to bed at night and promises to be there in the morning. As time goes by and the parents are always there, trust naturally develops. Normally, a mother takes a child to kindergarten and promises to be there at the end of the day to pick her up and then she is there when school ends.

Foster children do not learn trust as easily as other children do. As infants, they may not have been able to develop normal trust, and as older children, they have experience with bargains that were not kept. Each time you say something that you expect the child to believe, make sure you follow through. It is through repetitive acts of good faith that the child will learn to trust you.

Sometimes, part of your job is to help reunify the original family. It is important to try to reestablish the child's trust in his or her own parents. That may not be easy, but you should not make it any worse. If the mother forgets to show up, do not say, "I told you so." Tell the child that the mother is trying to do better.

Trusting the foster child is also something you will try to develop. At first you will not want to leave her unsupervised. Gradually you will allow the child some freedom, and if the child fails, you will keep her close to you again for a while.

PLAY

Many foster children have not learned to play. Their lives may have been so complicated that they did not have time, or there may not have been much play in their original homes. "The first time I went out to play ball with Jeremiah and I tossed the ball to him, he ducked. I had to roll it on the ground, for a while. I guess no one had ever played catch with him," said a foster father.

Foster children also may have trouble with the give and take of games. You may need to start with the basics. Try playing cards with the child if he is old enough, or build something with blocks. Let him follow your lead for a while. If the child needs more coaching in learning to play, try to get a teenager to volunteer to play with him. Learning to play with children of his age may take a little longer. You may select a neighbor or a relative who seems to play well with the child and arrange visits for a while. You will need to provide supervision and encouragement at the beginning.

When the child is playing around the house, keep an eye on him. Make sure the child is safe and he is not harming your possessions. Observe the way he plays. When you are sitting quietly later, comment on some of his actions and praise the things that you approve of.

CONFIDENTIALITY AND GOSSIP

As time goes by, you will learn a great deal about the foster child's family, and some of it may make you uncomfortable. In talking with a foster child, you need to develop a comfort level as her earlier life experiences are revealed to you.

At the same time, you need to be very careful about not sharing this information with others. Of course, the caseworker and the teacher need to know certain things, but your other children, your parents, and your friends should not know anything about the child's background. Coach the child to keep certain areas of discussion confidential between the two of you. If the child has had a difficult time in the past, she need not talk about the details with friends.

If you are in the same community with the biological family or if you are caring for a relative (kinship care) it is especially important to keep certain things confidential. "I don't gossip," is an appropriate quick reply to curious questions.

3

Foster Children as Part of a Foster Family

Foster care is exciting for most families. They say, "Never a dull moment in this business." Those parents who enjoy foster care often had foster siblings in their homes when they were children, and this large extended family has become a way of life. They look forward to a big crowd over the holidays. One said, "Thanksgiving was wonderful. I had Juanita and her new baby, Juanita's parents, her little brother who also used to stay with me and a big sister I never met."

Foster care should provide shelter for a child, but also should provide opportunities for the child to grow and change. The foster family will influence the foster child in significant ways. It will serve as a model for good behavior and loving relationships. At the same time, the foster child may influence the foster family as he or she brings cultural differences, new challenges, new emotions, and new successes to a preexisting family.

NORMAL FAMILY FUNCTIONING

Most families have certain features in common. In general, families work together in such a way as to benefit all members. There are certain family rules, such as always locking the front door. There are also family customs, such as who makes breakfast. Rules and customs have developed in order to strengthen the family.

Working together as a family may mean making sacrifices. "Our whole family gave up a lot, so that mom could go back to school. We were really proud of her, when she graduated," said a young woman. Families stick together, so that they have the strength of the family to support them.

In normal families, parents pay a lot of attention to the children. Parents try to provide opportunities for learning and growing. A game that is fun for a child may also be a learning experience.

On a day-to-day basis, decisions have to be made. In many families, children have some input into decision making. Difficult decisions are discussed at length, often at the supper table. Families must sometimes deal with problems. Certain occurrences are quite stressful to a family, such as a child failing a grade, an adult being fired, or an illness. In many families, everyone tries to support the member who has been affected.

In most families, if someone feels hurt, that will be quickly expressed and, if possible, the problem will be solved. Sometimes there is no good solution. Family members are generally willing to put up with some hurts in order to live within the family structure. Sometimes there is anger, but family members try never to harm anyone, emotionally or physically, as a result of their anger.

FITTING A FOSTER CHILD INTO YOUR FAMILY

If you have chosen to take in foster children and have completed the requirements to be licensed, you probably have a very nice home environment for a foster child. Still, there may be some challenges ahead. If your family has always worked together to benefit all members of the family, the foster child will add a new factor. The foster child may come from a different type of family, a different culture, or may have not had much family at all. It will take patience on the part of your own family to include the foster child in the process of working together.

If you have paid a lot of attention to your own children, you know that you will have to continue that level of attention with a foster child. You will try to find activities that will provide a learning experience for this child. The child may need considerable assistance and encouragement. One foster father said, "I took him to soccer, baseball, and basketball and he hated them all. You know what it turned out he liked? He liked to jog with me, after work."

Your family has already developed a way of making decisions. You sit together and try to figure out what will work out best for everyone. The foster child may be impatient with this process. He may just want to get what he wants and not spend time worrying about everyone else. Teaching him how a family makes decisions is extremely important. Be sure that you are fair with him and that his feelings are considered.

When there is a problem in the home be sure that the foster child is involved or at least aware of the problem. He may be extremely worried and may think the situation is worse than it is. If someone is ill, be sure and take the child aside to tell him what to expect.

The important thing is how you deal with the good times and the bad. Do you have some quiet suppers together, as a family? Do you bring up subjects that need to be talked through? Do you plan ahead, with the whole family, for outings and other activities? As good foster parents, you will see that opportunities for a child's growth are not missed.

OLDER FOSTER PARENTS

Commonly, foster parents are a little older than biological parents. Some foster parents are old enough that the foster children actually think of them as grandparents. If you are an older foster parent, you may feel a little out of touch with today's child rearing practices. There are several areas in which recommendations have changed.

First, note that children are raised less rigidly than in the past. Children tend to be allowed to select their own bedtimes, their own food for lunch, and their own clothes. The advantage of this style of raising children is that a child develops the ability to make decisions and learns the consequences of making unwise decisions. If the child stays up too late, he is tired in the morning. If you feel the need for a more regular routine, try to set up this routine together with the child and then help him stick to it.

A second area that may be different is discipline. In the past, more corporal punishment was used. If a child made a mistake, a spanking would be expected. At this time, it is recommended never to spank a foster child. Often foster children have been abused and they are very frightened by your anger. Discuss beforehand the areas that will require some obedience on the child's part and tell him the consequences. "I need you to be quiet in the car tomorrow, or else you will not be able to go with me the next day," is a way of stating your expectations.

In most cases, older persons are quite adaptable to caring for young children. As an older couple, you may have a steady income, good health, and few worries. You may have fewer stresses in your life now and be truly ready to relax and enjoy these children.

YOUR RELATIVES AND FOSTER CHILDREN

Ideally, you have worked out some of the areas of concern with your relatives before taking a foster child. One thing you need to discuss is confidentiality. Your relatives should not be told details about the child. They should not talk about the child with their own friends.

If you are going to provide a foster home, you will also provide a temporary set of relatives for the foster child. Your relatives may be unpredictable in their response to the child. Do not be surprised if the child warms to them and relates well to them. That is one fascinating aspect of foster care. It may turn out that your relatives are very important to the foster child. One former foster child said, "My foster mom's sister was kind of a role model. She was more relaxed than my foster mother was. She used to make me laugh. I learned a lot from my visits with her."

Elderly family members may have been somewhat dependent on your help, and such relatives may see the foster child as an intrusion on their time with you. You may want to schedule regular visits with such persons while the child is in school.

If you have disagreements with your relatives, be careful what you say. A foster child may have seen relatives physically fight. Now is a chance for the child to see how your family settles disagreements.

If you have adult children of your own, they may become involved with your foster children and they may actually become foster parents themselves. This is common, because whole families often take part in the process. One foster mother said, "My youngest daughter has her own child and now she and her husband have adopted Melanie, who was with me for a year."

WHEN FOSTER PARENTS ARGUE WITH EACH OTHER

You and your spouse may have occasional arguments. As it is very likely that the child has come from a home where conflicts resulted in physical fighting, your method of resolving conflict may be a learning experience for the foster child. Many foster children are fearful when their foster parents argue. They fear that a fight will break out, that one parent will leave, or that they may have to go to another foster home. Foster children often assume that they have caused the disagreement. If possible, try to comfort the child and tell her that all is well.

When you feel calmer, talk to the child about what happened. Tell her that you got really mad, but you did not want to strike out. Tell the child that you have been married for years, and occasionally you have to yell or cry a little over some issue. Be sure the child knows that you and your spouse continue to love and support each other and all the children in the house. "I hate these arguments with my wife, and Tiffany really freaks out," said a foster father. "Last time, she hid in a closet. The next day, I asked her if the yelling had scared her and she said it had. I told her that my wife and I expected to be married for a long time and that she could stay with us as long as she needed a foster home. I think she was relieved."

GETTING MAD AT A FOSTER CHILD

Most foster parents occasionally get angry with their foster children. You need to be careful in expressing your anger as these children often have had unpleasant experiences with angry parents. You may need to learn to count to ten or to take a few deep breaths before speaking. It may help to take a

moment to try to understand why you are angry and what the consequences of your actions will be.

When foster parents become angry with their foster children, they
should tell them why they are angry and then repeat their expectations. "I
get really upset when you leave dirty clothes on the floor. I expect you to
clean up after yourself," is an appropriate way to express your frustration.

Sometimes foster children try to make their foster parents angry. A good
foster parent will recognize when a child is trying to get negative attention
and will try one of two techniques. With a younger child, annoying behavior should be ignored and good behavior praised. With an older child, a
private conversation about trying to stop and think before acting may be
helpful.

Whether or not you spanked your own children when they made you
angry, you must never spank a foster child. Any physical punishment is unacceptable in foster care. If you have a child whose problems are so severe
that he or she needs to be physically restrained, professionals will help you
understand that process.

If you are having persistent trouble with your feelings of anger, talk to
the caseworker. It might help if the child has an activity to keep her busy
part of each day. Some agencies can provide respite care, where the child
goes to another home for short periods. On the other hand, it may be time to
change this child's placement.

Unfortunately, foster parents are sometimes accused of abusing foster
children and, indeed, sometimes they actually do abuse the children. Raising foster children is never easy, and it requires patience and self-control. If
you feel that you have reached your limit and before long you are going to
hit the child, call the caseworker. If you abuse a child, your days as a foster
parent will be over. More important, you will have negatively affected the
life of the child you have been trying to help.

CHILDREN FIGHTING IN THE HOME

Sibling rivalry, or disagreements between brothers and sisters, is a concern of most parents. Foster children will probably also fight and argue.
What do we know about sibling rivalry? Studies show that brothers and
sisters often fight to get their parents' attention. Other times a child may be
trying to get her own way, to get something of value, or just arguing for the
sake of passing time. Parents cannot hope to stop all arguing, but they can
encourage disagreements to stay verbal and not become physical.

Parents should try not to take sides in an argument. Suggest that the children try to think of a solution and you will tell them if it is acceptable. If it is
not, send them back to talk things over. As an argument turns into a nego-
tiation, it becomes a learning experience.

Experts feel that sibling rivalry may have some positive effects. A foster child, by getting involved in the arguments at your house, will learn how to defend herself verbally without physically fighting. This will be an important accomplishment to take back to the child's original home. She can say, "Here's how my foster sister and I avoided fighting."

Sometimes a particular child will become the victim at your house. Being hit and yelled at by other children can be a form of abuse. If it appears that a certain child always loses, sit down with the children and try to figure out what is going on. Consult the caseworker for advice. Sometimes foster children who are siblings need to be separated and placed in different foster homes.

Insist that children cannot hit each other in your home and insist on fairness. Praise them when they are cooperating and when they are playing quietly. When arguments begin among the children in the house, try to get them to negotiate. If that fails, use whatever form of "time-out" is comfortable for you. Separate the children for a period of time and set some ground rules for behavior when they do come back together.

THE QUIET CHILD

If a child is very quiet, she may be shy. You and your family should introduce such a child to new situations gradually. Try talking while you are doing something together, like cooking, or try talking when you are together in the car. Make sure that the rest of the family takes time to sit down and listen when the child wishes to talk. If she is especially comfortable with another relative, arrange regular visits.

There may be other reasons for the child being quiet, besides shyness. This child may feel "culture shock." She may feel quite different from you and your family. It may seem like no one understands her whenever she starts to talk. Also, the child may not understand what people are saying to her. Be alert for the possibility of deafness or speech delays.

There may have been problems in the child's past that led to shyness. She may have been raised in such a way that she was constantly criticized for everything she said. If that is the case, the child has been trained to keep quiet and it will take a long time to change that style of communicating.

Shyness may also be noted when the child is with other children. Friendships may have failed in the past or she may have had too many problems to have any energy to devote to friends. You can encourage friendships by having the child's friends at your house or taking them on outings. That will allow you to see how the child interacts, and afterwards you can make helpful suggestions. The child may be quite shy and quiet at school. The books and materials may seem new, other children may tease her, or the problem may be as specific as needing someone to sit with in the lunchroom. Special encouragement from you and the teacher will help her become comfortable at school.

Do not forget about safety issues, as this child may have difficulty asking for help. She needs to know your name, address, and phone number. Make sure she knows how to get to school and back. She should know not to get into a car with a stranger.

Shyness is a form of fearfulness and it will get better with your gentle encouragement. Your entire family may wish to work together to encourage the child. A foster child's shyness will gradually disappear as he or she gains trust in you and in your family.

FAMILY ACTIVITIES

Children take comfort from certain pleasurable routines. "My foster dad played gin rummy with me every evening for the two years I was there. I can still remember the way he would shuffle the cards. I was eleven and twelve during that time and I could beat him some of the time. Everyone else in the family left us alone for our game," one former foster child said.

Perhaps your family has some activity out of the home that is important. This may involve participating in sports or it may involve religion or music. Try very hard to get the foster child involved in this activity. She will be inspired by your family's enthusiastic participation. If you are not already a family that sings together or reads out loud, consider changing your ways. Try having each child select an article in the local paper to read at suppertime. Have one of the adults start a book with multiple chapters and read one chapter every night at bedtime.

In many cases, the foster child comes from a different cultural background. Think of ways that she can introduce her culture into your household. If possible, involve the biological family. There are many beautiful cultural traditions that you may not be aware of. The child's sense of importance, as she brings her own traditions to you, will be quite impressive.

After a foster child has left your home, try to maintain regular contact. Many foster families have at least one event every year to which they invite all their former foster children and their families. For most foster children, the experience in foster care will never be forgotten. As the years go by, you will need to catch up with the lives of your former foster children and they will need to catch up with yours.

CHORES

Whether or not children help with household chores differs from family to family. Foster children certainly should be expected to take care of themselves as best they can. If your children all make their own beds and pick up their dirty clothes, you should start with your foster child doing the same.

Do not expect more from him than from your own children, unless there is an age difference. In fact, you should expect less at the beginning. Praise the child for anything he does and expect him gradually to do more.

It is easier to insist that a child take care of his own needs than to get him to help with household chores. Give this some thought and when you begin with chores, handle this carefully. The foster child should not be required to do any more household chores than the rest of the children. Many former foster children talk about the "Cinderella" problem of feeling that they are expected to do too many chores.

Remember that he may never have done the things you expect. His life may have been chaotic, with little evidence of good housekeeping going on. The child may need to have a lot of hands-on guidance. Do each project together, having him or her do a little more each time.

An additional problem is that he may not be good at working independently. Even though the child understands the job, he may not be used to following through on the different steps. So as the child becomes more independent, keep an eye on him or her and provide encouragement. Praise him for doing the first few steps and be patient about explaining things over and over.

If this is your first foster child, think things through and then start carefully. It is possible to end up with a child who is so irritated over chores that he cannot proceed with the rest of the challenges of this period in foster care. Make sure the child learns to be helpful, but do not demand serious chores if he seems unwilling.

LATCHKEY CHILDREN

On the whole, foster children should not be home alone. Even older children can get into trouble or do dangerous things. The worst possibilities include starting fires, running away, or damaging your property. A new foster child should always be supervised. Take her with you, hire a sitter, or ask a relative or neighbor to be there. Then, very gradually, begin to make plans for leaving an older child home alone for short periods.

When an older foster child is home alone, make sure that the child knows how to reach you and how to call a neighbor. Leave a list near each phone with the phone numbers of the police and fire departments. Make clear what the rules are while you are away. If the child seems anxious or depressed, do not leave her alone.

What should be done if both foster parents work? This is a problem faced by many Americans. It may be all right if an older foster child is alone briefly, as when parents change shifts. Use your best judgment about that and consult with the caseworker.

Child care services are available for children of all ages. There are often programs at the school for school-aged children. If you have young foster children, a teenage neighbor may be able to baby-sit on a regular basis. Daycare, Headstart, and nursery schools often offer subsidized services for foster children. Be prepared to make phone calls to find out what is available, and then visit the program to see if it is right for your foster child.

DIVORCE AND FOSTER FAMILIES

Divorce occurs so commonly that foster children cannot be protected from it. Your family may already be a blended family with stepchildren or stepparents. You may be a single parent with or without a partner in the home. You may have started in foster care with a spouse and then become divorced while foster children were with you.

More than likely the foster child comes from such a family. Children in placement tend to come from single-parent homes and have had multiple half-brothers and half-sisters in and out of their birth homes. So the foster child may be familiar with broken homes but may also be familiar with the difficulties that can result.

If divorce is in your past, the important thing to demonstrate to a foster child is that you are not angry toward other family members or ex-family members. Try very hard to say pleasant things about your ex-spouse. Speak about him or her as an extended member of your family.

It is possible that you and your spouse will consider divorce while you are foster parents. It is important to talk to the caseworker if you think this is going to happen. There may be issues about where the foster child is going to be placed when the divorce occurs.

How you tell a foster child about this is problematic. Commonly, biological children feel it is their fault when parents divorce, and with foster children, this is even more likely. Someone may say, "They wouldn't have split up, if it hadn't been for Kyeesha." Even if the child does not seem to be worried about that issue, tell her repeatedly that your divorce is not her fault. Tell the child that you will both continue to love her and that she will be able to spend time with you both (if that is true).

Whatever happens, if foster parents divorce, the foster child will no longer be able to live with both parents. Try to keep the situation friendly enough so that the foster child can visit. Frequent phone calls will be helpful, especially if the child has to move to another foster home.

LEARNING THE ART OF CONVERSATION AT HOME

Most households are not quiet, so the first step towards a conversation is to turn off the television and turn on the telephone answering machine. Then, once it is quiet, you need to help teach a foster child how to engage in family conversation.

Foster parents should start by being good listeners. Settle back in the chair, have a look of interest, and respond occasionally with short questions. Praise the child for her contributions to the conversation. Laugh when you can and sympathize when it is appropriate. Encourage the child to tell you a story about something that happened during the day or a long time ago. Ask questions if the child does not complete the story. Sometimes you can develop a lesson from the story or suggest different endings. "What would have happened if you hadn't started to cry?" is the type of question that will encourage a child to think.

What should you talk about? The child needs to understand other people and why they do things. Help her talk about friends, your family, and adults in her life. Discuss activities of the day and the ways she interacted with other people. The child also needs to talk about her own family. She needs to figure out why they are the way they are. Remember how upsetting it is when people criticize your family and say as little as possible when the child talks about her biological family. Make neutral comments like, "Your mom has had a bad time" and "Your dad will probably do better."

Conversation may also involve you telling about events of your day, and these stories may also have a lesson. If your boss criticized you and you are feeling bad about that, discuss it with the child. Perhaps you need to change your work habits or change jobs. Children need to learn about adult problems and how adults handle their problems.

Be sure to share the happy moments of your day. If you stood in the sun during your lunch break and ate a hot dog and it was a wonderful moment, describe it to the child and ask her if she has had similar happy moments.

GAY FOSTER PARENTS

Some agencies will not place a child in a home where one or both parents are known to be gay or bisexual. In other situations, gay couples are raising foster children quite contentedly. Obviously, there are times when there is homosexuality and the agency does not know about it. With that in mind, what is the current feeling about homosexuality? Most people now feel that homosexuality is not a disease but a different lifestyle. Most people feel that a child's upbringing does not cause this lifestyle. It may actually be caused by differences in brain tissue or brain chemicals.

Many persons worry that gay foster parents will alter a child who would have been heterosexual, turning him or her into a homosexual. Although there is no evidence that this happens, this type of myth is quite persistent. Many heterosexual children have grown up in homes where the parents are gay, so this concern seems to be unfounded. Another concern is that homosexual adults will sexually abuse young boys and girls. The fact is that sexual abuse of children is relatively rare in homes with homosexual parents. Of course, abuse can occur in any part of society, and it is always unfortunate.

A good foster home has two happy, contented adults with time enough to pay attention to a foster child. As there is no evidence that homosexual parents cause any harm, there is no reason not to allow them to be foster parents.

TELEVISION

American families spend lots of time watching television. Sometimes people are engrossed in it, but often it forms a kind of background noise for adults. However, several aspects of television are problematic for foster children.

First, television may interfere with conversation and communication within families. Conversation is very important for a foster child to be able to make progress. Try to limit television to certain times and certain programs, then turn it off and turn on the radio, if you must have background noise.

Second, television may portray violence and stressful situations that are similar to the foster child's own experiences. If that is the case, it is important for the foster parent to be there to discuss it. Daytime talk shows often portray people having unusual, unsafe, or illegal lifestyles. Tell the child you understand that this may be bothering him and he is welcome to turn off the television. Try to monitor program selection better in the future.

The third problem is that so many families shown on television seem to be perfect. A problem arises and within twenty-five minutes it is completely solved. Here again it is important to talk to the child and tell him that life is not that simple.

The fourth problem is that television may provide an attractive escape for a foster child. Watching many hours of such entertainment will interfere with homework, with playing outside, and with reading for pleasure. Obesity in children seems to be related to excessive television watching.

There are a few times when television offers some opportunities for learning. A family may want to take advantage of these programs for a foster child. Also, a pleasant afternoon of watching a football game with dad may be a meaningful experience. For most foster children, however, television time should be limited.

PETS AND FOSTER CHILDREN

If pets are part of your life, that will not change when foster children enter the home. However, it is important to talk about safety. Pets can be harmful to children. Scratches and bites can cause infections. Make sure that your pet's shots are up to date. Also, you want your pets to remain safe.

Foster children have been known to feel sorry for pets and open the door and let them go free.

Pets have a relatively short life expectancy. You may have an aging or an ill pet. Talk to the child about it and tell her that you have been through this before. Tell the child how much you love the pet and that you hate to see the pet suffer. If the animal has to be put down, it may be just as well not to talk about the details. Just say you took the dog to the vet and the dog died. You should know that foster children are sometimes worried that they will be put down or put to sleep. Tell them that this is never done with humans.

Pets are loving and accepting, and a pet may become a true friend to a foster child. When the foster child leaves your home, he or she may have trouble separating from the pet. You may be able to arrange visits with yourself, the foster child, and the pet. At the very least, you may be able to send an occasional photograph of the pet to the child.

4

The Foster Child's Biological Family

Your foster child's own family is called the biological family. When a troubled family is brought to the authorities, the first approach is usually to provide services while the children remain in the home. Social workers and other professionals help these families to become stronger and healthier. If these approaches fail and a child is at risk of being harmed, the child is removed temporarily and placed in a foster home. After a period of separation, the child is generally returned home. About two-thirds of foster children return to their biological family within two years after they are removed.

The job of strengthening the child's family is up to the caseworkers, social service agencies, and the courts. Foster parents may or may not work directly with the child's birth family. If you are encouraged to get involved with the biological family, you will find it fascinating and challenging. You may find yourself sympathizing with the stresses in their lives and wanting to be as helpful as possible.

BONDING AND ATTACHMENT

Research shows that bonding occurs between infants and their parents even in many troubled families. This bonding is also called "attachment." When attachment has successfully occurred, children and their parents want to stick together. They recognize each other as family members and they feel that they have much in common. This attachment is part of the love that most children have for their parents.

Child welfare experts consider attachment very important. For that reason, most biological families are encouraged to maintain communication with their children during the period of placement in foster care. A foster child should always be thought of as part of his or her birth family.

In troubled families, mental health professionals sometimes feel that a parent and a child have not bonded well. This is not always the case with such families, and it is not appropriate for a foster parent to make such a diagnosis of "attachment disorder." In general, foster parents should assume that bonding has occurred and that there is love between parent and child.

Unquestionably, bonding also occurs between foster parents and a foster child. Mental health professionals feel that it is acceptable for such bonding to occur. Children have the ability to bond to more than one adult and such closeness should be encouraged. Foster parents become substitute parents and may, therefore, become very important adults in the lives of their foster children.

Separation is always difficult, after attachment has occurred. You might compare it to the discomfort of pulling off a bandage. Nevertheless, the discomfort of separation is not a reason to avoid attachment. Adults, as well as children, need to learn to form attachments without fear of separation.

WHAT BIOLOGICAL FAMILIES NORMALLY DO FOR CHILDREN

Families influence most children in positive ways. A child's parents make sure that the child remains healthy, gets an education, and stays out of trouble. Research findings on juvenile delinquency can demonstrate how parents normally keep their children out of trouble. From studies of juvenile delinquency and its prevention, it appears that the family plays an extremely important role. Although there is a tendency to blame the school or the neighborhood for a child's entrance into delinquency, a strong family can overcome difficulties with both.

What weaknesses in the family result in delinquent children? The answer is not in the problems of the family itself; rather, it is found in the relationship of the child and the parent. If the parent has not shown interest in the child, if the parent has not been actively involved in the child's life, then that child is at risk of getting into trouble. Families should be actively involved with their children. Parents or other relatives should be available to help a child make decisions and plan for the future. Children who grow up in a strong family will usually not get into serious trouble.

PREVENTIVE FAMILY STRENGTHENING PROGRAMS

If it is understood that children are protected against delinquency by having loving, caring parents, then how can professionals help troubled families change for the better? A preventive approach, which has been shown to have some real success, brings together families considered to be "at-risk" to learn how to be stronger and to function better. One method is to identify ten to twelve such families and plan a structured series of sessions. These are called "family preservation programs" or family strengthening programs. Sessions may be held weekly, each for two or three hours. The group works together under the guidance of a professional to understand ways to solve their problems.

Sessions in family preservation programs cover a variety of parenting subjects. There may be information about resources that are available, about drugs, prenatal care, or child safety. Parents may be taught ways to deal with their children (such as encouraging good behavior, planning the next day, or reading aloud). They will be encouraged to try different ways of reacting to their children and to each other. A very important component of such a program is role playing. A participant demonstrates a behavior and the group figures out better ways to deal with that situation.

Studies show that these family strengthening programs are quite successful. They are most effective if held in a setting in which the family is comfortable. The professionals who run the sessions need to be flexible in terms of scheduling and format. There should be incentives for families to become involved. Surprisingly, studies show that even when a family is required to participate in such a program by a judge or by probation, they still will show improvement.

If these programs are preventive, what about a family where troubles have already occurred? As foster parents, you are probably involved with such a family. Although there is not much research on such families and their response to family strengthening programs, there is reason to believe that such a family would also benefit. Talk to the caseworker if you feel that such a course would be helpful for your child's family.

GOALS FOR THE BIOLOGICAL FAMILY

In most cases, when a child is removed from home, there are multiple problems in the home. The caseworker or probation officer, with guidance from the judge, will determine which of these problems must be solved in order for the child to return home. Usually several goals are set. The foster child may also have individual goals to meet.

If a parent is an alcoholic or a substance abuser, successful completion of a rehabilitation program will be one of the goals. If child abuse or domestic violence has occurred, the perpetrator (abuser) may need to be removed from the home. If poverty has been a problem, the parent may need to get and keep a job.

Often family interactions have been unhealthy. Parents and children need to learn new ways to interact. The caseworker will guide the family through a series of sessions to learn how to handle problems, how to discipline children, how to control anger, and other similar issues. Foster families sometimes participate in these sessions. In some cases, foster parents work with the biological family directly to teach them better ways to get along. Parents of foster children may participate in formal programs held at outside agencies. These may be family strengthening programs or other types of programs to learn to get along better as a family.

VISITING WITH BIOLOGICAL PARENTS

Usually visitation arrangements are set by the court and handled by the caseworker. Birth family and foster family may meet soon after placement. The child may visit with his or her parents under supervision at the beginning. This allows the caseworker and foster parents to see the relationship in action and make suggestions. Other types of communication between the child and the birth parents are generally welcome, such as phone calls and letters. The child may need help with these activities from the foster parents.

As you watch the child interact with the family, try to think of some strengths that you see in the family and in the way they function together. You may notice that they are all kind to the toddler in the family or that the parents are quite interested in current events. When you talk to the foster child after the visit, bring up the strengths that you have identified and discuss them.

It is extremely important that foster parents are respectful of birth parents. Family visits are stressful and sometimes not satisfactory. Even if you are annoyed, it is best to say something neutral to the child. Tell the child that the next visit will probably be better and that you know he loves his parent(s). Besides making sure your words are respectful, be careful with your tone of voice and body language.

Unsupervised home visits may occur later. At these times, you may worry about the child's safety. Foster parents typically worry that the birth parents may be abusive, may not feed the child, or may not supervise the child. Talk these matters over with the caseworker.

If the child seems upset after a visit with parents, do not be surprised. Tell the child that you realize that these visits are stressful. Talk about how difficult it is to make any change, including the move from your home back to his own. Be sympathetic and let the child talk about his dreams, concerns, and sorrows.

GETTING READY TO GO BACK HOME

Toward the end of the foster care period, the biological family must show that they have the ability to provide food, clothing, transportation, and supervision for the child. All goals should be met, both for the family and for the foster child. Unsupervised visits will have gone smoothly and the visits may have lengthened.

If you suspect that the child will soon be going home, begin to talk about it. If you want to continue to be a part of this child's life and if the caseworker wants you to remain in touch, make some arrangements, such as, "I want to come to sixth grade graduation, so be sure that I get an invitation. I want to take you and your mom out for ice cream after it's over."

An aide or family worker may spend a few hours a week in the home immediately after the child is returned. The judge will order visits by the caseworker for a period of time after reunification to make sure all is well. In older children, probation may be involved after the child returns home.

Even though it appears that a child will go home soon, court dates may not result in a return home. If some problems remain, the child may stay in foster care for another period. Experienced foster parents are always ready for a child to return to them after a trip to court.

TERMINATION OF PARENTAL RIGHTS

Sometimes children are permanently taken from their parents in a process called "termination of parental rights." It is important to know that parents generally do have the right to keep custody of their children unless there is evidence of abuse or neglect. When the court removes a child from home against the parents' wishes, the state is acting as a parent under a legal tradition of *parens patriae*. After a child is taken away, parents have the right to have the child back if the situation improves.

If it appears that permanent separation may be necessary, the parent or parents are informed that the child will soon be taken from their custody. They are often given another chance to show improvement. These "second chances" may occur over several months. In most cases, when parental rights have been terminated, a foster child becomes adoptable. However, the time between termination and adoption may be as long as two to three years.

Avoid telling the child that you might adopt him, unless it is a certainty. Even a hint that you will adopt him or her may be quite harmful to his future mental state if such an adoption does not occur. At the point of termination of parental rights, another family or a relative may be considered appropriate for adoption and the child will be taken from you. Although it is best not to hint at possible adoption, it is usually appropriate to talk about seeing the child in the future. Begin to make arrangements, if you and the child wish, as soon as it appears that he might be leaving.

THE CHILD'S OWN BROTHERS AND SISTERS

Most judges try to keep siblings together when they enter foster care. If other siblings remain in the biological home, your child may be visiting with them when he sees the parents. Be sure and let the child talk about his brothers and sisters to you. He may miss them even when, in actual fact, their behavior may be part of the reason he has been removed.

Brothers and sisters may have come to your house together. In that case you can see how the siblings interact. Try to teach them about sharing. Tell them your rule about not hitting or being rough. Sit down with them when they disagree and try to let them talk it out. They may learn skills in getting along that will be useful when the foster children go back home.

Sometimes siblings are split up into multiple foster homes. In that case, the judge may have ordered visits. When the children visit together, you will probably get to know the other foster parents. Foster children may have half-brothers or half-sisters whom they do not know very well. You may discover that these youngsters have several different last names.

Older brothers or sisters may become involved with your foster child and begin to express an interest in helping raise this child. Making this type of connection for a child can lead to formal or informal kinship care and eventually to adoption, allowing the child to grow up with biological family members.

Foster children will watch your own children in action and learn from them. The rules should be the same for all children in your house. Sibling rivalry is best dealt with by using firm rules about behavior and by paying close attention to fairness.

HOW TO HELP A FOSTER CHILD SUCCEED UPON RETURNING HOME

If the birth family was somewhat chaotic, your foster child may have developed behaviors that actually made the situation worse. If the child was being neglected, he may have learned ways to make trouble in order to get attention. An older child with disruptive behavior may have been rebellious towards the family.

If getting the family back together is the goal, there are several approaches that will help the foster child and his family reach that goal. First, consider that the child is truly part of the problem, not just a victim. He is part of the family that was troubled, and if his behavior improves, it is more likely that he can successfully return home. Try to direct the child toward more positive ways of seeking attention. As you teach him to be more thoughtful and reasonable, the child will probably have a positive effect on his biological family.

During the period of foster care, the school may evaluate the child. If a learning problem is diagnosed, the child may be placed in a special classroom. In that case, when he returns home that placement will continue. Having success at school will make the child's home life more comfortable.

As you visit the doctor and the dentist, you may find various problems that can be solved. Correcting these problems will make the child's future a little brighter. Dental cavities, anemia, or lead poisoning are just a few examples of problems that affect behavior and can be corrected while a child is in foster care.

You and the caseworker may decide that counseling or visits to a psychiatrist would be appropriate. That will almost certainly be the case if there was abuse in the biological home. The social worker or psychiatrist will take many approaches to behavior issues that will be helpful as the family gets back together. Medication may be prescribed. Try to make sure that arrangements are made for continuing the medication and counseling when the child leaves your care.

BIRTH PARENTS WHO ARE INVOLVED IN SUBSTANCE ABUSE

The biological parents of your foster child may have been using illegal drugs, may have been abusing alcohol, or may have been involved in the sale of illegal drugs. All forms of substance abuse tend to cause significant problems within a family. Drug addiction and alcohol addiction are now thought of as illnesses, with periods of relapse. Rehabilitation programs have some success. Many persons need more than one opportunity to get off of drugs or alcohol.

If a parent of the foster child is a substance abuser, the judge may require rehabilitation in order to have the child return home. In other situations, illegal activity with drugs or alcohol may have resulted in incarceration for the parent. Persons who use illegal drugs or abuse alcohol have often developed habits of deception and of criminal activity. Foster parents often find it difficult to deal with such biological parents.

You may have a foster baby whose mother was a drug user or an alcoholic. Whether or not those babies are actually addicted, they are often fussy and jittery. Some communities now consider the use of drugs, alcohol, and even tobacco during pregnancy as a form of abuse. Such a baby needs extra nurturing from a loving and attentive foster parent.

With young children, you may be concerned about the child's safety as he or she returns home for visits. If you feel that drugs and alcohol are still being used in the home, speak with the caseworker. One biological mother said, "When you're using, you can't see the problems you're causing your children."

There are organizations for teenagers who have addicted family members. Such groups meet and discuss ways to understand and deal with these issues. An older foster child can benefit by that kind of interaction. It may offer a resource for that child after he returns to the biological family.

In addition, a foster child whose parents are drug users may need to be evaluated for the HIV virus. Talk to the caseworker and see if a test has been done. If not, talk to the doctor or clinic. Testing for HIV is essential in order to arrange for appropriate and timely treatment.

BIRTH PARENTS WHO ARE MENTALLY DISTURBED

One feature of adult mental illness is that such persons often are not able to form close relationships or to show love toward their children. Children of severely mentally disturbed adults may be taken away for periods of time and placed in foster care.

Schizophrenia is such a severe psychiatric problem. Afflicted persons may seem distant and confused; their thought processes may not be logical. Usually schizophrenia can be kept under control with medication. If you are dealing with a schizophrenic parent who seems more confused than usual, that person may have stopped taking his or her medication. Depression, in an adult, causes sadness and feelings of hopelessness. Depression and suicide can go together. Try to be as understanding as possible with such persons and encourage them to seek professional help. If medication has been prescribed for depression, encourage the person to continue taking the medicine.

A foster child whose biological parent is mentally disturbed may be able to go back home for periods of time. Caseworkers should maintain some connection with these families and, if the mental condition becomes worse, the child may need to be removed again. Some such families receive respite care in which a child is removed for short periods of time on a regular basis.

Older children who have mentally disturbed parents may understand that the problem can be inherited. Allow the child to discuss this issue and help him or her find resources that might be helpful.

BIRTH PARENTS WHO ARE VERY YOUNG

Many foster children were born to teenaged mothers. Very likely, such a mother had her first child at age fourteen or fifteen. She may have had other children soon after. In the foster care system, you will see the unfortunate results of adolescents having children.

The stories of very young women who get pregnant are somewhat predictable. "Ginny was fourteen and her boyfriend was twenty-two," said a foster mother. "He left her as soon as she said she was pregnant, and then her parents threw her out of the house. She was only in ninth grade, but school was over for her. I guess she got involved in drugs and prostitution. Now I'm raising two of her kids. Gosh, it's sure a sad story."

In the case of a foster child whose mother is quite young, foster parents may be extremely helpful in teaching parenting skills. Very often the young mother is invited to visit regularly to learn about raising children and managing a household. Such a young woman should take every opportunity to get more education, such as a high school equivalency degree. She should take parenting classes, stay away from drugs and alcohol, practice safe sex, and focus her attention on her child. Foster mothers can work with these young women in a positive, friendly way. They can cook and shop together, and foster mothers can provide valuable information to the young biological mother.

Foster parents may help establish connections with the foster child's father or with the extended family of a teenage mother. Part of helping such a young woman is helping her understand that the infant's father and her own family members may provide resources for her and for the infant.

BIRTH PARENTS WHO ARE ILL OR WHO HAVE DIED

A foster child may come to you as a result of his or her mother's death. When young women die, the cause was probably violence, drug-related, or HIV/AIDS. It is important to learn as much as you can about what actually happened.

With HIV/AIDS and other terminal illnesses, the mother may have been ill and the child may have remained at home. The child may actually have helped take care of the mother. The child may have missed school, missed opportunities for sports, and missed the companionship of other children during that time. The child may be angry with her mother for leaving her. That is a common reaction whenever a youngster loses a parent.

If the mother died a violent death, did this child witness the event? The child may be quite disturbed as a result and also may be fearful that there will be more violence. If the child did not witness the event, she has undoubtedly developed a mental picture of what happened. You may want the child to talk about this to you, so that you can help her understand.

A foster child whose mother has died can benefit by getting to know other members of her biological family. Try to help the child establish or reestablish ties with the birth family. Also listen to her concerns about the death of the mother and try to help her adjust. You may need to get professional help for the child.

BIRTH PARENTS WHO ARE IN JAIL

Many of the hundreds of thousands of Americans in jail or prison are parents. In most cases, the parent who is incarcerated is the father. If the father of your foster child is incarcerated, he may be able to write or call the child. He may want to stay involved with that child's life, and, in most cases, child care experts feel that this is appropriate.

Sometimes foster children have parents who have gone to jail because of crimes the children saw committed. Or the crime may have been perpetrated against the child, such as with physical or sexual abuse. These are extremely uncomfortable situations, and a foster family will need the guidance of professionals for ways to handle such a child.

If a parent who is in jail would like the child to visit, that may be arranged. It will be extremely stressful for a child to see his or her parent in jail. Even entering the jail is stressful for children. However, in most cases the parent will eventually be released, and parent and child will interact again at some later time. So these visits, painful as they may be, are useful in keeping connections among family members. Some jails and prisons have special programs to allow children to visit with their incarcerated parents. If you feel such a visit would be helpful, talk to the caseworker.

NOT WANTING THE CHILD TO RETURN TO THE
BIOLOGICAL HOME

Often foster parents express the feeling that the child should not return home. At the same time, the fact is that most children love their own parents and want to live with them. Children old enough to understand are often quite angry that they have been removed from their parents. Many foster children feel that they are part of the birth family and they yearn to return to it. Former foster children often remember wanting to go back home.

Although foster parents often regret that a child has to go back to the biological family, it is important to try to remain optimistic and to remember that people can change for the better. "All four of those kids were taken away because their father was having problems with alcohol," said a foster father. "There was no food in the house, and I really think he was abusive. Now he is a regular part of Alcoholics Anonymous and he has a job. Should those kids go back? Yeah, I guess so."

The point is that people truly do change. They may not look perfect, but the whole family deserves a chance to live together again. As a foster family, when you send such a child back, your home will be available for temporary placement of another child.

BIOLOGICAL FAMILIES WITH CULTURAL DIFFERENCES

Many families have specific features that differ from those of your family. Biological parents may be hearing impaired, non-English speaking, or mentally retarded. In these situations, it may be challenging to make a foster child entirely comfortable in your home.

A common situation is that a Caucasian family takes an African-American foster child. Of course, skin color is only one aspect of this child. In many other ways, she may have a lot in common with a Caucasian family. However, the foster child may face problems of prejudice and discrimination at school or in the neighborhood. Your extended family may be unhappy about the presence of this child in your home. Also, an African-American biological family may be unhappy about the placement of their child in a Caucasian home.

It is always good to talk about differences in race, religion, and ethnicity. The child needs to remain part of the culture she came from throughout her stay with you. Introduce the child to your lifestyle, but at the same time try to adapt to her interests, holidays, clothing styles, manner of speech, and any other differences that may arise. One special concern is a child who comes from a bilingual home or a non-English-speaking home. It is important to retain the child's language skills in the original language so that she can speak with the biological parents.

If a child has moved in and out of several foster homes, she may truly not know what her ethnic background is. That is particularly true if the child started out with a mixed background. "I've had a couple of foster children who didn't know if they were Black, Hispanic, or Bosnian. They'd been all over and lived in all kinds of places. I tell them they're just Americans and that's a good thing to be," said a foster mother.

HOLIDAYS AND OTHER EVENTS AND THE BIRTH FAMILY

Nothing is as important as getting families together for special events. Holidays are quite special and there are cultural aspects of family holidays that cannot be replaced by a foster family. Although you should encourage visitation during religious and non-religious holidays, this is also a period of stress and worry. "She said she'd pick me up on Thanksgiving and she never came," said a foster child.

Weddings and graduations are important family events. It is fine for foster children to participate in your family activities, but it is also important that they be part of their own families' lives. Encourage the caseworker to arrange appropriate visits.

There are times of trouble for all families, and the child may need to feel a part of these troubles. Terminal illness or death, trials and going to jail are just a few examples of the times a child should not be left out of a family. A child who is excluded from an activity may have an incorrect idea about what occurred, and fantasies can be more disturbing than the real events.

KINSHIP CARE

Kinship foster care is taking a relative into your house as a foster child. The term "informal kinship care" means that the child is not officially a foster child. Both formal and informal kinship care are very popular, especially in African-American families. About one-quarter of children in foster care are placed with relatives. Kinship care is encouraged because the child remains part of his or her own biological family. Also, it is easier to arrange visits with the birth family and reunification is often simpler in these cases.

However, there are areas of concern with kinship care. If the entire extended family is weak or troubled, the situation may not improve for the child. Grandparents are often the foster parents and they may have health problems because of their age. Also, if an abusive or neglectful biological parent remains nearby, the child may continue to be mistreated.

Kinship care may result in long-term foster care. In that case, the child will stay with the relatives until he or she grows up. Another possible outcome is that the relatives may take over guardianship of the child. Adoption is generally made available to such families, if the parents' rights are terminated. In many of these situations the placement will continue to be subsidized until the child grows up. Some older children do not wish to be adopted, but do wish to remain in the family. Judges are fairly flexible in establishing living arrangements for such children.

MORE THAT YOU CAN DO TO HELP FAMILIES REUNITE

Some foster parents become quite intensely involved with the biological family. These foster parents may participate in family visits and may have the child's parents in their own home for visits. This usually involves working closely with the caseworker as part of the team. It is extremely satisfying to see a foster child's birth family begin to function better.

"Shared family foster care" involves actually placing a parent or parents into the foster home. This is fairly common when an adolescent foster child has a baby. She may remain in the foster home and raise the baby there with the foster parents' assistance. In other situations, such as with mentally retarded parents, the entire family may live in a foster home for a few months.

Biological families may be willing to learn from a foster parent. Trips to clinics or trips to a child's school activities can all be learning experiences for birth parents. If the caseworker does not suggest involving birth parents, ask if it is appropriate. If the birth mother does not want to participate in these activities, perhaps the father or another relative would be willing to participate.

Even if a foster child is never reunited with the birth family, the time spent working with the birth family will benefit the child. The bond of parent-child attachment may have been quite weak in the past and your efforts may strengthen this bond.

5

Abuse and Neglect

About half of the children in foster care have been removed from birth parents that abused or neglected them. In actual fact, almost all foster children have suffered some neglect in the past. There are five types of abuse and neglect: physical abuse, sexual abuse, emotional abuse, physical neglect, and emotional neglect. Even though judges remove many children from abusive environments, others remain at risk. It is estimated that approximately 2,000 children die each year in the United States at the hands of their parents or caregivers.

A child who has a history of maltreatment often fails to develop normally. Certain behavior problems and emotional problems are common in these children. They often have trouble forming relationships with adults and they often do poorly in school.

Foster parents may be quite disturbed by the stories these children tell. There are ways to help such a child cope with his or her past, and there may be ways to teach the children to avoid abuse in the future. The judge may have put a plan in place to reduce the abusive nature of the family in order for the child to return home. For abusive biological families, counseling and other programs may help prevent more abuse in the future.

TAKING ABUSED CHILDREN AWAY FROM THEIR HOMES

In the 1970s it was determined that an abused child could and should be removed from an abusive home. State laws were developed to address this concern. At the present time, laws in each state vary in the definitions of abuse and neglect and the way the courts deal with it.

The courts have struggled, through the years, with issues of parents' rights. It is assumed that, in general, families have the best ability to raise their own children and should be allowed to do so. The state has the power to take a child from his or her parents only after establishing that the family is unable or unwilling to raise the child. The doctrine of *parens patriae* presumes that children are unable to take care of themselves and that the state has the child's best interests at heart.

Physical abuse and sexual abuse are fairly clearly defined, even though they may be difficult to prove. Severe abuse may result in the abuser going to jail, and in that case, the child may not be removed. Physical neglect, emotional abuse, and emotional neglect are harder to define and harder to prove. There are cultural issues that must be considered. Children are seldom removed from the home solely because of neglect. Instead of removing the children, the judge and authorities will arrange for services to be provided in the home.

When a family goes to court because of abuse or neglect, the children may not be removed. The judge may require certain activities and a plan for social workers to monitor the safety of the child. If a child is removed from his or her parents, most judges will recommend placement in a relative's home, if one is available. This may or may not be formal kinship foster care. If the child must be taken from the home and a relative is not available, the child will enter the foster care system. The law requires immediate plans for reunification or termination of parental rights. This is called "permanency planning" and is required by federal law.

CHILD PROTECTIVE SERVICES (CPS)

Child Protective Services is part of county government in most cases. Each CPS unit consists of social workers, lawyers, and supervisors who are specialized to handle issues of child abuse. Phone calls reporting abuse generally go first to a hot line at the state level and are then handled at a local level by CPS workers, sometimes together with the police.

When a call comes in, the CPS worker asks for as much information as possible. Anonymous calls can be acted upon, but with some difficulty. The workers generally visit a home within twenty-four hours of a call. CPS workers begin to keep a record as soon as a call comes in. At some point they determine the accusation to be founded or unfounded. If an accusation is unfounded, it is assumed that abuse did not occur, and the record is erased. If an accusation is founded, the CPS worker will stay involved. He or she may make unannounced home visits, supervise homemaker aides, and arrange counseling and other activities. In some cases, CPS workers recommend immediate removal and that is ordered by family court.

Abusive parents tend to respond better to someone who tries to help them rather than to someone who threatens them with removal of their children. Experienced CPS workers learn to be sympathetic and concerned when dealing with such parents. They offer substantial help, such as food and clothing. They make suggestions about improved parenting practices rather than simply demanding changes.

CPS workers generally have a thankless job. Parents usually do not want their children removed and children usually do not want to leave. If the court does not choose to remove a child and there is further harm to that child, the CPS worker may feel responsible.

DISCOVERING AND DOCUMENTING ABUSE

Although a child of any age can be abused, abuse occurs most often with toddlers. They are noisy and active and parents cannot reason with them. Family members who have impulsive tendencies will hit them to try to quiet them. The children are too small to hit back or to protect themselves. Often the abusive person is the mother or father. Another common situation is abuse at the hands of the boyfriend of the child's mother.

When a child is brought to the emergency room with a history of frequent fractures or other signs of physical abuse, the doctor may choose to call Child Protective Services and keep the child until the situation is clarified. This may involve several hours of attention by police and social workers. Laboratory tests and X rays may be required, to document the extent of abuse or neglect.

Abused children may or may not admit to being abused. They are often embarrassed by the situation and by their helplessness. An abused child may feel guilty and believe that he or she caused the abuse. Such children often know that admitting the abuse will result in removal from home. In addition, their parents may have threatened them and told them not to tell. Most children want to preserve their privacy and preserve their biological families.

There are also cultural issues. In impoverished homes there may be fighting and aggressiveness among various family members. Sometimes abused children feel that what has occurred is normal. Talking about what has happened may feel like giving away family secrets.

ABUSIVE FAMILIES

Abuse and neglect seem to result from various family stresses, such as poverty, alcohol, drugs, and unemployment. About one-third of child abusers were abused themselves. In about half of the homes where children are abused, there is violence between adults, which is called domestic violence.

The abuser is often the father or the mother's boyfriend. The man may be unemployed and frustrated by his lack of financial security. He may be unable to manage his anger, be unreasonable in his expectations regarding obedience, and have a tendency to use alcohol or drugs. For various reasons, mothers who live in such a household find it difficult to take the children and move out. There may be several young children in the home, making such a move difficult. The mother may not be able to afford to leave. Further, she may be afraid that the man in her life will be angry if she leaves him.

Mothers and fathers in abusive households tend to expect obedience from children. They are not patient with childish behavior and they hit a child expecting that child's behavior to improve. Such a parent is verbally demanding, yelling rather than reasoning with a child. The abuse typically ends when the child is old enough and big enough to fight back successfully. An abused child who grows up and remains in the home often abuses the younger children.

Sometimes the mother is responsible for the abuse or neglect. In such cases, drugs or alcohol may be a factor. A woman who is looking for illegal drugs or needing money for alcohol has little time to devote to children. The children may be neglected and may be left alone for periods of time. When the mother becomes frustrated she may hurt them.

When a child is injured and needs to go to the emergency room, abusive families may delay taking the child and may offer vague explanations about the extent or cause of the injuries. They may seem unsympathetic and uncaring. A parent may indicate that the child fell off a sofa or wandered into the street rather than accepting responsibility for the abuse or neglect.

CHARACTERISTICS OF ABUSED CHILDREN

Psychiatrists say that children who have been abused have difficulty attaching to adults and have little trust. They seem unemotional and they may not relate well to other children. Young children will tend to have disorganized play. Language skills may not be well developed and the children tend to do poorly in school. Studies show that children who have been abused tend to have difficulty in making friends.

Certain resilient children seem to do well even though they have been abused. High intelligence, good school performance, high self-esteem, and understanding that abuse was a result of the parents' frustrations and hopelessness are all helpful factors.

Some foster children have permanent injuries resulting from abuse by the biological family. These injuries may be severe, such as brain injury resulting from being shaken. Other injuries are somewhat disabling, such as burn wounds. The foster child needs to know what to say if there are questions about scars or other signs of past injuries. With anyone except medical or legal persons, the child may want to say he or she does not know how it happened. The foster parents should say as little as possible to their own friends and relatives about the details of past abuse.

FEARS OF ABUSED FOSTER CHILDREN

For most abused children, fear has become a normal part of their life. They are fearful of the abuser, afraid that no one will believe them, and fearful that the abuse is their fault. It appears that many abused children actually deny the abuse is happening. This seems to be a type of self-protection.

Foster children who have been neglected may seem quite worried about getting enough food and other necessities. Such a child may hoard food or may eat very quickly. In the past, the child may have stolen food and other needed items as a survival tactic. The child may seem selfish when dealing with other children and learning to share may be difficult.

An abused child entering a new foster home may be nervous about the possibility of continuing abuse. A statement such as, "We never hit our kids or our foster kids," may be comforting for such a child. Similarly, the child may need to be reassured with each new situation that no one will hit him. He may be fearful of strangers. These fears may persist for many months and tend to be worse at night than during the day.

A child who has been sexually abused may be unexpectedly flirtatious or extremely withdrawn. There may have been a prolonged series of sexual encounters in his or her biological home. Such a child may be quite frightened at night and need constant reassurance that there will be no sexual contact in the foster home. Foster parents need to be extremely cautious about touching or hugging a child who has been sexually abused. Also, be sure you prohibit sexual contact of older children or other adults in the home regarding this child.

SUGGESTIONS FOR FOSTER PARENTS OF ABUSED CHILDREN

Children who have been abused or neglected need to begin to get some satisfaction out of life. They may need help in various aspects of development that have been missed, such as toilet training or learning to read. Avoid teasing such a child for his or her behavior, looks, or attitudes. Try not to criticize or scold. Set reasonable rules and insist that the child follow them. Establish reasonable consequences if rules are not followed.

Such a child needs to be praised when he or she does well, and the benefit of such praise is significant. "Nobody had ever told me I was a good kid, until I came here. Now they tell me that a lot and sometimes I almost believe them," said a formerly abused foster child. Success may come in small steps with such a child. Watch closely for small successes and praise the child as often as you can.

Foster children should be encouraged to ask lots of questions and to try to understand things. They should be allowed to have opinions and the family should respect their opinions. A child who has been abused or neglected will learn a lot from watching your own family interact.

Hugging and touching may be problematic. Hugging preschoolers is usually acceptable. With older children, avoid having them sitting on adult laps or kissing adults on the lips. Find other ways to express warmth with a genuine smile, a laugh, or a touch on the shoulder. Children can be encouraged to sit next to an adult on a sofa, but more contact than that may start sexual feelings in a child that should be avoided in a foster home.

SPECIFIC TYPES OF PHYSICAL ABUSE

State laws vary and judges vary in their definition of abuse. Abuse exists if there is an injury and if there was intent to injure. Occasionally, there is clear evidence of abuse, as when a child has a broken bone and a witness was aware of the intent to injure. However, more often, the situation is less clear.

Fractures, or broken bones, are common results of physical abuse. There may be multiple fractures in various stages of healing. One type of fracture, a spiral fracture, results from a twisting injury and is often due to abuse. The abuser commonly is a parent, who jerks a young child up in the air by the arm in anger. Often abusive families have an inappropriate explanation regarding a fracture.

A scald burn occurs when a child, usually a baby, is put into a bathtub with excessively hot water. Another burn that is commonly seen in abused children is a cigarette burn. Most other childhood burns occur as a result of inattention rather than intent to injure. Bruises are common in abused children. Areas involved are usually different from those of a normal active child and may include the back, buttocks, or upper arms. A child who has been beaten with a belt or an electric cord may show characteristic skin lesions.

Various types of head injuries are common. A skull fracture usually results from trauma with a heavy object. The "shaken child syndrome" results from shaking a child so hard that the inside of the head is injured. Brain damage may be severe with such an injury. Putting a pillow over a child's head can result in suffocation. In an autopsy this cannot be distinguished from Sudden Infant Death Syndrome (SIDS).

SEXUAL ABUSE

Sexual abuse occurs more often in girls than in boys. Although definitions vary, rape and any kind of sexual intercourse between an adult and child is sexual abuse. Any use of a child for pornographic activity is abusive. In most cases, sexual abuse is suspected when a child discloses such activity. The perpetrator is usually an adult male in the home, either the father, the stepfather, or the mother's boyfriend.

Most pediatricians agree that it is difficult to prove sexual abuse by examining a child. In extreme cases, there may be bruises around the vagina or anus. Pregnancy in a young girl is evidence of abuse, and sexually transmitted diseases, such as gonorrhea, indicate abuse.

Children who have been sexually abused in the past demonstrate some behaviors in common. They may be quite shy and frightened around strangers. Or the other extreme may occur and the sexually abused child may show quite explicit, provocative behavior. The child may talk quite freely about sexual activity that he or she has seen or participated in. Girls who have been sexually abused may have self-injurious behavior such as cutting or marking themselves. They also have a high incidence of anorexia and bulimia. Sexual abuse apparently causes some girls to become prostitutes.

If a child has been sexually abused and that becomes known while the child is in your care, you need to advise the doctor and caseworker about this. The child should be tested for sexually transmitted diseases. The caseworker will decide if further legal steps must be taken.

You should tell the child, based on his or her age, that sexual activity should not occur between children and adults. You will not allow it to occur in your home. Masturbation is acceptable, if it is done in private.

THERAPY FOR A CHILD WHO HAS BEEN SEXUALLY ABUSED

A foster child who has been sexually abused needs to feel that he or she is in a safe environment and that abuse will not occur in your home. She must know that some action has been taken regarding the abuser.

A social worker, psychologist, or psychiatrist can provide therapy for a sexually abused child. Such a therapist should have experience with this type of work. The child should be allowed to talk about her experiences with the therapist. If the child is quite young or quite disturbed, play therapy may be used, allowing the child to act out situations rather than talking about them.

As a child talks about past experiences of sexual activity, the therapist will help the child to understand what happened. The child must be made to understand that the sexual situation was not her fault. By talking about it with a professional, the child should begin to put the experience behind and move on with his or her childhood.

A child who has been sexually abused needs to learn what is appropriate sexual behavior and what is not appropriate. You can help by pointing out situations in the newspaper or on television where sexual activity was not appropriate. If the child is old enough, he or she may be able to learn ways to prevent the abuse from happening again. You and the therapist may help the child become more assertive. It might be quite useful for her to learn self-defense or karate. The child should not feel guilty about the past, but she should face the future with as much confidence as possible.

As a child becomes an adolescent, therapy may focus on understanding the youngster's own sexuality. Starting to date may be disturbing for a child who has been sexually abused. As a foster parent, you may be quite helpful as you listen to this child's concerns and offer suggestions.

FAILURE TO THRIVE, NEGLECT, AND EMOTIONAL ABUSE

These forms of abuse and neglect are difficult to define. Sometimes it appears that parents, in such an abusive or neglectful family have limited parenting skills. They either ignore the child or shout at the child, but they do not mean to harm the child. Judges generally do not remove a child from his or her biological home because of one of these forms of abuse.

"Failure to thrive" means that a young child does not grow well. This may occur because the child is not fed adequately, but it can also be caused by lack of love and attention. A young child who is not gaining weight may be hospitalized and evaluated to make sure there is not a medical problem that can be corrected. If no medical cause is found, the child will probably gain weight while in the hospital.

A child who has been neglected has not been given adequate care. There is physical neglect, medical neglect, emotional neglect, and educational neglect. A neglected child may be thin or droopy, may have developmental delays, and may not have good health habits. He or she may not attend school regularly. Routine medical attention and immunization may not have been provided.

Emotional abuse occurs when parents yell, harass, and threaten children. It is hard to prove that this is occurring if this is the only type of abuse. This type of childrearing results in children who do not get along well with other people. They have heard only criticism, never warmth.

Children who have been neglected will usually respond well to a period of foster care. These children may be less disturbed and less angry than children who have been physically or sexually abused.

SENDING ABUSED CHILDREN BACK TO THEIR BIRTH HOMES

Even when abuse has been proven, children who have been placed in foster care are often sent back to their biological families. The abusive person may no longer be in the home. In other cases, the abuser may remain in the home, but he or she may have successfully completed a preventive program for such persons.

The child's biological parent may have demonstrated to the court that he or she has changed. The mother may be off drugs. The father may now have a home and a job. Because child abuse is often a result of poverty, efforts to improve the family's finances will help a mother get her child back. The mother may have married, moved in with her own mother, or made some other arrangements for assistance. In these circumstances, the judge may feel that the child will be able to live in safety.

There are some common frustrations for foster parents regarding sending children back to such homes. First, there is no guarantee that the child will not be abused again. Judges try to determine if the home is safe, but they understand that there is a certain amount of risk. Second, the legal system does not allow the child to have the right to make a decision. Until a child is an older teenager, the judge will not pay much attention to his or her wishes.

Some foster parents become quite insistent that the child's biological home is not safe. In some areas, foster parents are allowed to go to court and speak to the judge about their concerns. Local foster parents' organizations may be helpful. If it seems inevitable that the child will return home, discuss future safety issues with the child. Perhaps you can review ways for the child to avoid getting hit and encourage the child to find after-school and summer activities out of the home. Help the child understand whom to call for help and when to call for help in the future.

HOW TO MAKE A CHILD LESS ABUSABLE

In many chaotic families a young child needs to yell and carry on to get attention. Then, when he gets attention, the parents criticize or hit him. Such a child is seeking attention in negative ways. "There he goes, he's doing it again. That's when he's expecting to get smacked," said one foster brother. You can be quite helpful if you develop ways for the child to change this attention-seeking behavior. A foster child should ask politely for your attention and should get a quick response from you. The child will be encouraged to continue this type of behavior if you respond quickly and warmly.

Children who have been sexually abused may appear to be quite provocative. Do not encourage this behavior. Tell such a girl that she should not kiss and hug people who are not in her family. In your home, discourage cuddling and sitting on laps, especially between foster daughters and foster fathers. Talk to the child about not allowing touching in certain parts of his or her body. Exceptions to the rule include health professionals.

If you do not participate in visits with birth parents, you will probably hear about the visits. Listen carefully to the things the child tells you. Identify ways the child may make his parents angry and help him to change. The child should not feel that the abuse is his fault; however, the abuse may decrease if he changes certain behaviors.

You and the child, together with the caseworker, should discuss ways to deal with future abuse. If the child returns home and, at some point, the abuse starts again, what should this child do? You may want to encourage a young child to call you, so that you can contact appropriate authorities. An older child should have clear instructions about dealing with abuse, if it happens again.

THE CYCLE OF ABUSE

Studies show that about one-third of abused children grow up to abuse their own children. It is also known that adults who are violent have often been abused as children. Foster parents can help make sure that this cycle of abuse does not continue and that this child does not become abusive as he or she grows up.

The child should have opportunities, in private, to discuss the abuse that has occurred in the past. He may want to talk to the caseworker, to a psychologist, or to the foster parents. Abused children should be taught that abuse occurs because of stresses, such as poverty and unemployment. The child should not feel any blame for the abuse.

Studies indicate that a child who can attach to an adult and form a relationship will probably not become an abusive adult. A foster child needs a mentor to talk with and to help get rid of some of the anger and frustration. Establishing such a relationship with an adult helps a child to learn trust and develop good self-esteem.

Families with domestic violence and abuse tend to raise violent children. In such homes, older children often hit younger children. Children who are hit may respond by hitting back. This is another cycle of abuse, and you can help the child learn not to hit other children. You need a firm rule that there should be no hitting in your house, then reasonable consequences should be established and enforced.

The cycle of sexual abuse is also potentially problematic. A boy who was sexually abused when he was young may force sexual attention on others as he becomes older. Foster parents who are raising a sexually abused teenager will want to pay close attention when the youngster shows an interest in dating. A person who forces sexual attention on others is a sexual perpetrator or a sexual offender. There are professionals who specialize in dealing with sex offenders and special programs are available.

ALLEGATIONS OF ABUSE AGAINST FOSTER PARENTS

If a foster child feels that he or she is being abused in your home and reports that abuse to the authorities, there will be an immediate investigation. Sometimes such an allegation is true and sometimes it is not. In either case, the situation can become quite tense. Abuse in foster homes can take the same forms as abuse in biological families. Often it occurs because another adult has entered a foster home. "Everything was fine with little Janie until my daughter's boyfriend moved in with us," said a foster mother. Ideally, caseworkers should make frequent visits to every foster home to make sure that there are no harmful changes in the child's environment.

Foster children may be argumentative and disobedient, and such behaviors may result in an adult getting so frustrated that he or she hits the child. Another problem is the foster child who is seductive and sexual around adults in the home. A foster parent may have a weak moment and give in to that seductiveness. Thus, physical abuse and sexual abuse happen, from time to time, in foster homes.

Neglect is also possible as payment is low for these children. A foster parent is generally given a check for the child and not asked to account for how the money is spent. If the foster parent chooses to spend that money on himself or herself, the child may not get necessary food and clothing. This type of problem would occur less often if caseworkers visited foster homes on a regular basis.

False allegations of abuse are the greatest fear of many foster parents. Foster children may know that accusing a foster parent of abuse will stir up a lot of activity, bring a lot of attention, and usually will result in a new placement. If you feel that your foster child is unhappy and if he or she has been complaining about your treatment, take action. Call the caseworker. Consider ways to make the child's life more satisfactory or consider recommending a change in placement.

6

Newborns and Infants

Some foster parents become experts at taking care of babies. The foster babies may have been abandoned at birth or may have been removed by the authorities at a young age. Whether placement is temporary or permanent, the baby deserves a home where there is love, attention, and knowledgeable care.

Do very small children understand what has happened to them? That is a hard question to answer. It does appear that normal babies bond with their mothers. Although babies sent into foster care may miss that bonding experience with their biological mothers, research suggests that a nurturing figure, such as a foster mother, may make a big difference to the baby.

Children who enter foster care usually come out of poverty, and children born into such a family are likely to be premature and have other problems. Thus, these are often not normal newborns or infants, and they may need special care and attention.

HAVING A FOSTER BABY IN THE HOME

Mothers have very strong maternal feelings towards their own newborns. With a foster baby, foster mothers often report that they have some of the same maternal feelings. At the same time, foster parents may become overwhelmed because a foster baby may be fussier than a biological baby, may not have good sleeping habits, and may be difficult to handle. Family members may need to help with the baby because of fussiness and crying.

Although sometimes a baby will enter foster care immediately after a normal delivery, often the child will have spent a lengthy time in the newborn intensive care unit. Some infants have had a trial home with the biological mother and that trial has failed. So, even if the baby is quite young, there may have been a difficult period for that child before coming to your house.

For parents and babies, feeding should be a quiet time to be together. You should try to create some pleasant moments to sit down to be with the child. Try to make feeding time restful for the baby and for yourself. Remember, the newborn period lasts for only a few months. It is a very important time for the baby to have attention from a nurturing caregiver. Try to cut back on any unnecessary outside activities. Spend any extra time or energy you have cuddling the baby or singing songs to the baby. Whatever this child may have already missed, you will accomplish a lot by providing a little extra attention in the first few days or weeks at your house.

Other children, your own or foster children, may react in unexpected ways to a baby's arrival. The baby may take an enormous amount of your time and the other children may be jealous. They may miss the attention that they are used to receiving from you.

HELPING THE BIOLOGICAL MOTHER OF A YOUNG BABY

The baby's own mother may be quite involved with the foster parents. If this is the case, you will not only be raising a baby, but you may be helping a young woman cope with motherhood. It is a challenging, but satisfying, responsibility. In most cases, when a newborn enters the foster care system, the goal will be reunification, bringing the child and the mother back together. Try to talk to the baby's biological mother and father about the rewards of parenting. Talk optimistically about the child's future and positively about the baby. Tell them that you love the child, but you will be happiest if, in the end, they are all living together.

Often, foster mothers have an opportunity to try to teach the young mother how to care for the child. Biological mothers may be invited into the foster home on a regular basis to learn how to feed and diaper the child, bathe the child, and cope with crying and fussiness. If a baby is going to return home, there are things to consider. Will the biological mother need child care so that she can work? Does she have a crib, car seat, high chair, and other necessities? You may be able to help the mother and the caseworker in obtaining these items.

If it appears that the baby will not end up returning home to the mother, it is still important to try to establish a good relationship between the baby and the biological mother. The caseworker and the judge will decide if such visiting is appropriate. In general, children benefit from knowing about their mothers whether or not they eventually reunite.

CHILD CARE, BABY-SITTERS, AND PRESCHOOL
FOR FOSTER CHILDREN

You need to have appropriate baby-sitters for an infant, so that you can get to outside events. Be sure the person is comfortable and competent with babies. As the child grows older, you may want to look for a Headstart program, for child day care, or for a nursery school. Talk to your caseworker about subsidized programs that might be available for this child.

In many states there are regulations about day-care centers and day-care homes. Investigate the regulations in your state, and then evaluate the facilities according to those rules. Contact other parents to make sure it is a safe and supportive environment.

A handicapped child may qualify for special attention at home, in a regular preschool, or in a day-care center. The caseworker should be able to help you get these services. If you need other help, contact to the child's doctor, the local health department, or your school district.

AIDS AND THE HIV VIRUS

As foster children usually come out of poverty, foster parents naturally worry about whether the child might have had contact with the AIDS virus (the human immunodeficiency virus, or HIV). In most states, the caseworker is required to give you any available information about a child's health, including the results of HIV testing.

In larger cities, there is a realistic possibility that a foster child will have had a mother who was HIV-infected. Such a child may not become infected, but the virus is sometimes transmitted to the child. If transmission has occurred, the baby's blood tests will be positive within the first few days or weeks of life. If it is found that a baby's HIV test is positive, the child will need to see a physician right away. Most likely the child will be sent to a specialty clinic where these problems are handled regularly. Medication may be indicated and the child will be followed with frequent clinic visits.

If your foster baby is HIV-infected, ask the doctors if there are any particular precautions or whether the baby needs any special care. In most cases, universal precautions will be recommended. That means wearing gloves if you are to be exposed to the baby's blood and washing your hands especially carefully after changing the diaper.

Also talk to the social worker or counselor in the clinic. Ask this person about how to handle your emotions, how to talk to the biological family, and what to tell your own family. Babies who are HIV-infected almost always have an HIV-infected mother, so there will be additional concerns as you deal with the biological family.

Children with this condition need lots of love and affection. They may or may not have a long life ahead of them. Whatever the outcome, they are likely to need special medications, treatments, and tests for the rest of their lives.

ABUSE AND NEGLECT IN INFANTS

It is hard to understand why adults mistreat children, especially why they mistreat babies. However, mistreatment is a fairly common reason for removing children from their parents. One form of mistreatment, neglect, is almost always a result of poverty and a difficult home situation. With abuse, the other form of mistreatment, the abuser may be the stepfather, father, mother, or mother's boyfriend.

Neglect is a form of mistreatment that involves not providing routine care to a child. Young children can be neglected by not being fed, by not having clean diapers and clothes, or by not being loved. Neglect can cause failure to thrive, which means that a baby or young child does not gain the weight that is expected. If a baby has failure to thrive, tests should be done to make sure that there is no physical illness. When this type of neglect has occurred, there is usually an attempt to provide counseling and guidance to the parents. If the child fails to gain weight while remaining with the parents, there may be hospitalization and there may be placement in a foster home.

Physical abuse of young children, which is sometimes called battering, can take several forms. It occurs most often during the "terrible twos" when children, even in normal households, can be annoying. Head injury is the most serious form of abuse. It may result from actually hitting the child, shaking the child (shaken child syndrome), or dropping the child. In any case, a child with a head injury may have changes in consciousness and changes in ability to think and function. Gradually, with good care, these children improve, but some brain damage may be permanent.

Other forms of abuse are unique in very young children. Broken arms may occur when someone jerks a toddler by the arm. Abused children may have multiple fractures in various stages of healing. Scald injuries may result from bathing an infant in excessively hot water; this is a form of neglect. When a family appears to be abusing a child, social workers and caseworkers try very hard to keep the child safe. Placement in foster care is common, but not required. Abuse can be fatal if the situation is not altered.

A young child who has been abused has had a very bad experience with life. As the child matures, there is healing. The physical problems may disappear, but the emotional problems may persist. The caseworker may consider counseling when the child is old enough to benefit.

RAISING FOSTER BABIES

Foster parents of a young baby are the most important caregivers in the baby's life. The approach used in handling a foster baby may make an enormous difference in the development of the child.

Babies understand, at a very young age, when you are encouraging them. Always comment on good behavior. Use smiles, praise, and hugging to indicate your satisfaction. If the positive aspects of behavior are encouraged, unwanted behavior like fussing and crying will tend to disappear.

As the baby begins to move about the house, let the child explore as much as possible, keeping safety in mind. Young children find many things interesting. Encourage a baby to show you interesting things she has discovered. As language develops, let the child talk about her exploration.

Do not physically punish a baby, especially a foster baby. If an infant is irritating you, she is not doing it on purpose. If you are quite frustrated by a foster baby, you should get some help. In general, if a child is doing something you want to discourage, ignore the child. Do not show pleasure or displeasure. If you consistently ignore a baby with certain behaviors, that behavior gradually will begin to disappear.

As a baby grows old enough to understand rules, make sure that the rules for the child's behavior are simple and clear, appropriate for her age. Do not argue with a baby or yell at a baby. If a child's behavior is unsafe, such as running in the street, take her out of the street. Watch the child more closely, so that she cannot get away, then encourage and praise the child when she stays with you.

Foster parents often have fairly strict schedules, and in general that is good for young babies. They tend to do well if there is a routine structure to their day. Bedtime, mealtimes, and activities should all occur at about the same time each day.

Take a few moments to think about raising this foster baby. By encouraging behavior that you like, you will help this child grow up to be well behaved. Try to get agreement about parenting practices with all the adults who are involved with this baby. Talk with your family, the caseworker, and the biological family and continue to encourage them to be consistent.

DISCIPLINE WITH BABIES, INFANTS, TODDLERS, AND PRESCHOOLERS

Most experts agree that, with very young babies, there is no such thing as spoiling. Babies need almost unlimited attention and they respond well to that attention. Yet, as a baby grows up, he or she needs to learn limits. The child needs to understand the meaning of the word "no."

Most experts would suggest never spanking or punishing a very young child. Any parent might be tempted to spank when a young child runs in the street. However, there is no evidence that spanking is a good way to discipline a child, and it is especially inappropriate for a foster child. Try to be firm and set high expectations. Make sure young children understand your rules for safety and behavior as much as they can. Plan to supervise all young children carefully so that they are safe.

Even a young child will want to find out what your limits are. "How much will she let me do?" he might think. When a toddler begins to explore limits with you, do not give lengthy explanations. Pick the child up, sing a song, or otherwise distract him. Picking up an infant who is misbehaving is an early form of time-out. Time-out is simply a matter of giving the child a chance to think things over for a few moments.

As the child gets a little older, time-out may mean putting the child in a certain place to think about his behavior. With young children, it may mean moving the child away but in the same room. "See that bottom step? That's my time-out spot. It's eight feet from the kitchen table. When I tell Sam to sit on that step, his behavior usually improves," said one foster mother.

AGGRESSIVENESS IN YOUNG CHILDREN

If you have not had young children in your home for a while, you may have forgotten how they behave. If your foster child, still a toddler, is hitting and biting, this may be essentially normal behavior. On the other hand, this may be worse than normal if he has learned to be unusually aggressive in the biological home. Talk to the caseworker and the child's doctor.

If a young child comes to you acting very aggressive, give this child a lot of ways to use up his energy. Take the child outside for walks and games. Consider a play group for short periods of time, so you can watch him with other children. A structured day-care setting or Headstart may be quite appropriate for socializing this child if he is old enough. Try very hard not to react to aggressiveness by spanking the child or yelling at him. If he hits another child or a pet and you respond by spanking, that encourages the behavior that you are trying to stop. It results in a cycle of hitting and "hitting back."

This child may have come from a troubled family and may return to one. Any way you can improve his behavior by preventing aggressiveness will help him and the family in the future. As the child becomes old enough to talk, tell him how much you like him or her when he is being kind and helpful to others. Tell the child stories or read stories that involve children learning to get along.

Try to cut down on television watching. Children are very impressionable and the violence and anger on television may become a way of life. Many television cartoons, quite attractive to young children, are especially violent. Children may model their behavior on what they see on television. This is especially worrisome with foster children, who may not have good strong family values. Computer games can involve violence and you may also want to limit this activity.

INFANTS BORN TO DRUG ADDICTS AND ALCOHOLICS

A newborn may go into foster care immediately after birth if the mother is addicted. In many communities, a drug test on the mother is done at birth, and if the test is positive, the baby is removed until the mother completes rehabilitation to the satisfaction of the judge.

A baby of a drug addict or an alcoholic mother tends to have multiple problems. The child is likely to be born small or premature. Babies whose mothers are addicts tend to be very fussy, to cry a lot, and to be fidgety. "Fetal alcohol syndrome" is a condition resulting from alcoholism during pregnancy. Babies with this syndrome have unusual facial features, short stature, and mental retardation.

The children of addicts are likely to remain smaller than average as they grow and to demonstrate low intelligence and poor coordination. Such a child may qualify for an early intervention program and will probably benefit by such a program, which may include speech therapy and other services. A preschool or nursery school will also be helpful when the child is old enough.

There is no proof that the newborn baby of an addict is addicted. Neither is there convincing evidence that the child of an addict is likely to become an addict unless he or she grows up into the lifestyle of the parent. All studies indicate that a warm and affectionate foster home can be important for such a child.

FEEDING A FOSTER BABY

A newborn baby coming right from the hospital will be started on formula. It is best to continue on the same formula until she is at least six months old. The formula should have iron in it. Premature babies and allergic babies may be on special formulas. A newborn will take two-to-three ounces per feeding and should be fed every three-to-four hours. The amount will gradually increase to six-to-eight ounces at six months of age.

If you take in an older baby, there may have been no consistent feeding pattern. Buy formula with iron and begin feeding the baby. The baby will tell you when to stop and when she is hungry the next time. Begin to establish a pattern based on the child's responses. When the child is four-to-six months old, she can be started on cereal. After six months, many babies go on regular milk and whole milk is recommended. As there is no hurry to have the baby eat solid food, it should be introduced in such a way as to make feeding a pleasant experience for her and for you. Give the baby a little cereal from a spoon to start with. Baby food should be added gradually, as tolerated. Try to wait several days before starting each new food.

Vitamins and iron are not usually needed as they are added to the formula. If your water supply does not have fluoride, have the doctor give you a prescription for a fluoride supplement. Do not put the baby to bed with a bottle. Try to keep her upright for one hour after feeding.

SLEEPING, COLIC, AND FUSSINESS FOR NEWBORNS

Most newborn babies sleep many hours, waking up from time to time and then going back to sleep. Normally, when a baby wakes up, the caregiver's presence is reassuring, and the child goes back to sleep. For a foster child, there may not have been a loving face to relate to in the past. Therefore, the foster child may not have established a clear pattern of sleeping, and may wake up often during the night. Foster mothers who take young babies are used to a lot of fussiness for the first few days or weeks. They consistently comfort the child, using body contact, gentle motion, and soothing songs.

A baby who has colic cries persistently for no obvious reason. The crying tends to occur around suppertime and the baby may seem quite upset. For a foster child, this type of fussiness might be partly a result of difficulties in the past. Make sure the baby does not have an ear infection or some other medical problem causing pain. Ask the doctor if a change of formula might help. If the baby has colic, no medication will stop the crying. The problem will probably continue until the child is four or five months old. You may be able to find a relative or neighbor who can help take care of the child occasionally. Rocking the child or carrying him about with you may help.

DOCTOR VISITS AND IMMUNIZATIONS

Take a baby to the doctor as soon as you can. If possible, take the baby to the same doctor or clinic that this child went to in the past. When the child is measured and weighed, write down the data. Ask the doctor if the weight is adequate. The baby may need to get more immunizations and if immunizations are behind schedule, extra visits may be necessary. Make sure you have a complete record of immunizations.

Ask about any special concerns you have regarding this child and write down the answers. Put all information from the doctor into the folder you are keeping for the child. If this baby goes back home or to another home, the record should go with her. Discuss the child's development. If you and the doctor agree that there are significant delays in language or motor skills, consider a referral for an evaluation. The clinic will be able to help you with appropriate referrals. Let the caseworker know of these plans.

Also, make sure you know how to get medical help at night or on the weekends and that you know what hospital to go to in an emergency. Make another appointment for the next visit before leaving the clinic.

SAFETY

If you have not cared for a baby for a while, take note of the new recommendation for sleeping position. Newborn babies should sleep on their backs or should be propped on the side. Sudden infant death is more likely to occur when a baby is put face down in the crib. Very old cribs may be unsafe, but those built after 1974 are considered safe. Do not give a baby a bottle in bed.

By five or six months, babies will learn to roll over and then be able to move around. Keep cleaning supplies, medications, matches, and lighters locked up or up high. If there are weapons in the house, make sure they are up high, in a locked cabinet, and unloaded. Do not leave a baby unsupervised. Watch the floor to see that there are no coins, buttons, or pins. Make sure your valuable knickknacks are out of reach. If you are in an older home, consider having the home tested for lead. Be sure that the bath water is not too hot. It is recommended that the hot water in your house be kept below 120 degrees.

Many children have been hurt by falling out of walkers, so it is best not to use one. If a walker is used, make sure it has a wide base and keep the child away from stairs. When traveling in the car, the baby should always be in a car seat. Make sure the car seat is attached according to manufacturer's instructions. Make sure swimming pools are not accessible to babies or children.

IRON DEFICIENCY ANEMIA

This problem can occur in the first year of life if the child is not given iron-fortified formula. Research shows that anemia can actually decrease a child's intelligence. Most doctors check for anemia at around one year of age. If there are questions about diet or about behavior, a blood test for anemia should be done. Iron deficiency anemia is treated by giving an iron supplement.

CONSTIPATION

Constipation is defined as having dry, hard, bowel movements that may require straining or cause pain. Even if bowel movements occur only every other day, the baby is not constipated if there is no straining. If there is extreme straining or if there is bleeding, check with the doctor. You may need to add fiber to the diet and increase fluid intake. Switching formula or stopping dairy products may be suggested.

There is a congenital defect called Hirschsprung's disease in which constipation occurs because of a birth defect in the large intestine. It cannot be recognized without testing. If constipation is a persistent problem, that should be considered.

VOMITING AND DIARRHEA

If a newborn sometimes spits formula back up after a feeding, that may be a normal occurrence. Wait a few minutes and try feeding the child again. Sometimes vomiting indicates a child has a viral illness. If so, the child will be droopy, have a fever, and probably have diarrhea. If the child seems ill, wait a few hours before starting feeding again. Try water or juice when you start and gradually return to a normal diet.

Reflux can cause persistent vomiting. That occurs when the stomach contents roll back up into the esophagus and out of the mouth. It helps to feed the child in a sitting position and keep her upright for an hour after feeding. Some pediatricians suggest that you thicken the feedings by adding cereal.

Projectile vomiting is very dramatic and the child seems to vomit large amounts. This may be caused by "pyloric stenosis," which means a valve in the stomach is too tight. The condition is diagnosed by a doctor and treated with surgery.

Diarrhea occurs when a child has many loose, runny bowel movements. If diarrhea continues for more than a few hours, watch the child for signs of dehydration. A dehydrated child produces very little urine and is listless and droopy. If these signs develop, call the doctor. Otherwise, give plenty of fluids and wait for the problem to pass.

RASHES

Diaper rash may be present when the child first comes to you, especially if there has been neglect. You should change diapers frequently, keep the area clean, and put protective cream on the skin. Call the doctor and see what kind of cream is recommended.

Milia is a rash with small whiteheads on the face of newborns. It does not need treatment. Eczema causes a scaly rash on the ears, elbows, and knees. Hydrocortisone cream can be tried. Cradle cap causes an oily, scaly area in the scalp. Some mothers use baby oil on the scalp to treat it.

Birthmarks usually require no treatment. A strawberry hemangioma looks like a slice of strawberry attached to the skin. These usually disappear in the first few years of life. A salmon patch is a dark reddish area on the forehead, eyelid, or scalp. A Mongolian patch is a brownish area on the back or buttocks and can be mistaken for a bruise.

TALKING AND LANGUAGE DEVELOPMENT

Babies start to vocalize or make sounds as soon as they are born. At about a year of age, they begin to use actual words. Typically a one-year-old child says four words, although variations occur often. Young children generally understand some things that they cannot yet say. At that stage, they often have nonverbal communication, with gestures and sounds. Some toddlers who have not learned to talk, can communicate well with gestures.

Children learn to talk by imitating people around them. A foster child may be slow to learn to speak because of neglect. Such a child will probably catch up quickly in a good foster home. Make sure to talk clearly and repeat commonly used words. Sing for the child and read aloud. These activities stimulate speech development.

If a child seems to have delayed language and speech does not improve quickly, talk to the doctor. There may be a hearing problem that can be corrected. If delays seem serious, have the child referred to an early intervention program for an evaluation. If a child is found to need speech therapy, attend some of the sessions. Pay attention to what the speech therapist is doing and ask how you can get involved. It will be helpful if you do the same, or similar, activities at home.

A child with speech delays will benefit from a preschool program when he or she is old enough. Talk to the elementary school in your neighborhood and see what programs are available. See if there is a Headstart program or a day-care program that your foster child can attend.

HEARING AND VISION PROBLEMS

Hearing problems are hard to recognize in the first few months of life. You can experiment a little by whispering to the child from the side and watching for a response. Vision problems may also be hard to recognize. Some babies have an eye that turns in or some other obvious abnormality of the eye. Diminished vision may only be noticed when the child is old enough to move about, and you see that he bumps into objects and sits near the television set.

If you suspect that the child does not hear or see well, speak to the child's doctor and see if special tests need to be arranged. Hearing aides and glasses can be used in very young children and may make a tremendous difference to a child's development.

A foster parent who identifies such a problem can help the child start to deal with it. Children may need special equipment and special training if they are severely vision- or hearing-impaired. Try to make sure the child is enrolled in programs that will be helpful. Many of these special programs will be available to the child wherever he or she goes in the future.

PHYSICAL DEVELOPMENT—SITTING AND WALKING

Normally a child rolls over by six months, sits by nine months, walks with assistance by twelve months, and walks alone by fifteen months. There is some variation in these milestones, but a delay of several months is a cause for some concern.

Foster children may have delays due to the way they have been raised. The child may not have had appropriate encouragement to develop well. If physical delays are caused by birth defects or mental retardation, the child may need occupational therapy or physical therapy.

If a foster child seems a little slow in motor milestones, the whole family may help. Spend time encouraging the child, getting down to her level. Use a lot of body language and be very enthusiastic. If the child has the potential to be normal, she will catch up within a few months. Remember how you applauded when your own child first stood up. Use that same enthusiasm to help foster children learn to walk and run.

If physical delays continue and there is little improvement, speak to the doctor. Blood tests for anemia, lead poisoning, and thyroid problems should be done. Evaluations need to be arranged with appropriate specialists. If no medical problems are found, the doctor can help you with further suggestions and referrals. Occupational therapy and physical therapy may be helpful.

SOCIAL DEVELOPMENT

Foster children tend not to develop socially at the same rate as other children unless they remain in one foster home from birth. Bonding between a mother and child is important, and if that was missing, the child will be slow to show interest in others.

By the second month of life, a normal baby recognizes his mother's voice and looks around to find her. When he recognizes the mother, the baby will smile appropriately. If these reactions are not occurring in a foster child, that may be because of a long hospitalization early in life. It also may occur because the child first went to a neglectful home. In very young babies, you can see improvement in social skills as you spend time holding the baby and talking and singing to him.

With some foster babies, social development continues to lag. The child does not seem to respond to caregivers or to others. This may be due to severe neglect or abuse in the past. Or it may be due to mental retardation or to some other developmental problem. If you are concerned about social development, talk to the doctor. See about having the child evaluated. In the meantime, continue to be especially loving and attentive.

PROBLEMS WITH TOILET TRAINING

You may have a foster child who is old enough to be toilet trained, but has not yet attained that milestone. Someone else may have started the process and you need to continue. Talk to the child and find out how much he knows or understands. If the child is not old enough to talk or able to talk, he probably cannot be toilet trained. Some children are fearful of the toilet and some are just not ready.

If a child is over the age of three and you feel he needs encouragement to start using the toilet, get him to agree to try giving up diapers. Establish regular times for the child to sit on the potty. Find quiet activities to distract him. Expect toilet training to be more challenging for a foster child than a child of your own. Be patient and persistent.

Some children can learn to urinate in the toilet, but bowel training is delayed. This is especially common in boys. Speak to the pediatrician about this problem if it persists.

EARLY INTERVENTION FOR INFANTS WHO ARE SLOW IN DEVELOPING

The federal government has mandated that services must be provided to children who are handicapped. Such services are available for youngsters between the ages of zero and twenty-one. For babies and preschoolers, this program is called "early intervention." The child will be evaluated and, if there are physical or mental delays, a plan will be developed. Therapy and other help should be provided in a convenient location. Services may include physical therapy, occupational therapy, speech therapy, and educational assistance. There is no charge for these services.

In some states, there may be problems accessing these early intervention programs if a child is not with the parent. Your caseworker should be able to help make appropriate arrangements. Studies have shown that only about half of the foster children between the ages of zero and three who qualify for early intervention are receiving services. Getting your foster child enrolled in an early intervention program will be quite beneficial.

If a program is arranged for your child, the professionals will request the presence of the foster parent at some of the sessions. It would be a good plan to try to include the biological parents in these sessions also. A strong, consistent early intervention program will help a young child succeed when that child enters school.

7

Six- to Twelve-Year Olds

Between the ages of six and twelve a child generally develops a personality and a sense of right and wrong. During this same time, individual strengths and weaknesses can be identified. For children who grow up in a family, the family is a strong influence and guides the child in certain directions. For children in foster care, the caseworker and foster family must provide guidance for this type of development.

Children at this age are away from home much of the day. Besides school, they may be involved in sports, in lessons, and in religious training. There may be many hours spent in play activities that are not structured. The child will learn to function in a world away from home, learning to deal with other children and with other adults.

During these middle years of childhood, children have little ability to think theoretically. They may not be able to understand both sides of an issue. They cannot realistically imagine their own future.

Adults help very young children by praising their good behavior and ignoring their bad behavior. Adults raising teenagers have long, thoughtful discussions of all the possible consequences of a behavior. During the middle childhood years, there is a transition from one style of parenting to the other.

BUILDING SELF-ESTEEM IN FOSTER CHILDREN

Self-esteem is the ability to respect oneself. Poor self-esteem results from a lack of love, an insecure environment, and not being treated with respect by one's parents. These may be exactly the features of your foster child's upbringing. What are ways to encourage such a child to feel better about himself?

A foster child needs to hear more about his good qualities than his shortcomings. He should be praised for making wise choices and not simply for being obedient. "You did fine when you shoveled the driveway next door, because Mary can't do it for herself," is encouragement for having made an independent decision. This type of encouragement may be quite helpful for a child who has often been criticized. The child will learn to respect himself, as you express your respect for him.

When a decision needs to be made by the child, talk it over. Have him think through choices and the consequences of those choices. If possible, let him make the final decision. Afterwards, ask him if the decision worked out. If it did not, ask what he learned. Either way, praise the child for taking the time to think things through. A child gains self-confidence as he continues this process of thinking things over when he is not with you. Ask the child about decisions he made when he was away. Use the same approach by asking him what was learned and praising him for thinking things through.

When the child has had a success, even a small one, recognize that success. Make a poster or take a photograph. Put it on the refrigerator and continue to point it out as a record of the child's success. Praise him for strengths you have seen, such as honesty, helpfulness, or persistence.

BEING HELPFUL TO OTHERS

Psychologists use a term "prosocial behavior" for behavior that is helpful to others. A foster child may feel that life has treated her so unfairly that she does not need to care about other people. However, helpfulness is a very important adult behavior that a foster child should learn in your home.

When a child is quite young, parents encourage the child to share. This involves sharing physical things, like snacks and toys, and also sharing ideas and plans. People of all ages may find sharing difficult, but it is a very basic trait that should be encouraged. It may be a new and difficult concept for a foster child, so keep your expectations reasonable.

As children become older, they should understand that if a family member becomes ill, they should respond with sympathy. They should offer to bring a glass of orange juice, to turn down the television, and answer the telephone. Sympathy and an expression of concern, when appropriate, are signs of prosocial behavior.

The equivalent of the Golden Rule should be something that all children are taught. They should learn that kind actions on their part will result in kindness from others. For younger children, find books or tell stories that will illustrate the benefits of being kind to others. For older children, remember to point out that pleasant, thoughtful behavior is quite helpful for the child's ability to get along with others.

In some cases, the child's own biological family may not show much sympathy for the child who is in your care. In that case, the child may be angry. Help the child deal with a lack of prosocial behavior in his family. It is always helpful to tell the child, "Mom is trying hard and she's got a lot of stresses in her life." Having this attitude toward everyone will help the child to be successful long after he or she has moved away from you.

GETTING ALONG WITH OTHER CHILDREN

Besides getting along in a family, the foster child will need to get along with children in the neighborhood. It is important to help foster children learn to make friends and keep them. You cannot always protect a foster child from trouble, but you can try to predict trouble and teach him ways to prevent it. Also, if the child does report problems in getting along with others, you can be comforting and at the same time help him learn ways to get along better.

Some foster children are quite shy around other children of their age. Do not be surprised if your brash and bouncy foster son or daughter is quite aloof with other children. Be patient and tell him to be patient. Continue to point out his strengths and help the child use those strengths to make friends.

Instead of being shy, some foster children may seem thoughtless and rude around other children. Your foster child may ask other children questions that make them uncomfortable. He may annoy other children by teasing them. These may be personality traits that the child has developed in the past. Encourage him to be more thoughtful when with other children.

Your foster son may be a fighter. If he comes from a home or neighborhood where physical fighting was common, he needs to know that there are new rules that apply not only to your house but also to the neighborhood. If he hits someone, there may be consequences and he needs to know that in advance. Teach him ways to handle his anger, such as counting to ten.

NEW EXPERIENCES—GETTING MORE SOPHISTICATED

Foster parents may be surprised to find that a foster child has never been to a restaurant or to a sports event. You will need to introduce each new experience, to describe things before they happen, and to prepare the child for any special behavior requirements. Afterwards, praise the child for the things he or she did well.

A foster child is like a foreign exchange student. You have an opportunity to show him a new way of living. Make sure that the child is exposed to a variety of cultural activities, such as a museum, a craft fair, or a circus.

Most of these activities are inexpensive and nearby. Prepare the child and afterwards ask him what he learned. Gradually increase your expectations for the child, expecting him to accept new things better as he grows older.

It is best if a foster child tries a new experience with you and the family, not when he is out with others. Try to make sure that you have exposed the child to places and situations before he goes alone or with friends so as to spare embarrassment and frustration on the child's part and your own. As a foster child is introduced to activities that are challenging for him, set a goal of staying just a few minutes. Then, if the child does enjoy the activity, you can stay longer. Remember that he may have a fairly short attention span and if an activity requires a lot of concentration, possibly he should stay home with a baby-sitter.

GOOD MANNERS

Foster children may not have learned to trust and respect authority if they have been raised in a chaotic environment. When you teach a child good manners, you essentially are teaching respect. When a child treats the authorities in life with respect, that person reacts by trying to be helpful. Examples of such authorities are a teacher or a caseworker.

Foster children may have had contact with law enforcement in a variety of ways. The child may have a very negative view of police officers or probation officers. With a young child, find stories to read or tell stories about the helpfulness of such persons. Help the child interact in an appropriate way, whether or not it is an important interaction.

With medical persons, social workers, principals, and anyone else who may deal with a foster child, teach the child to look at the adult and to answer questions to the best of his or her ability. When foster children return to their biological homes, their ability to speak up when they go to see a social worker or a doctor may be extremely important.

From time to time, ask your foster child to call and see if the library is open or make other such appropriate phone calls. When a call is more difficult, practice ahead. Have the child learn to call the caseworker, as that may be very important in the future.

Watch the foster child as he or she reacts to your family members, neighbors, and other adults. Coach the child about shaking hands, about appropriate voice quality, and what to say when you enter or leave a house.

ADULTS AS MENTORS FOR FOSTER CHILDREN

A mentor is an adult or older child who can become a friend for a foster child and help the child to grow and develop. Although a foster parent may become a mentor for the child, it is often someone outside the home who fills this need.

Ideally, such a person will continue to be involved with your foster child after the child leaves your home. You may or may not recognize mentoring, even while it is going on. Many adults look back on someone who was important in their own childhood. "My Aunt Mary was always there for me. She wanted me to get out and do something with my life," said a teacher.

Also, many adults remember a child who was important to them. "I'm so proud of Alex. He's working in New York City now, but sometimes I read his name in the local paper. I spent a lot of time trying to get him to straighten up," said a minister, regarding a foster child he had known. Such an adult is remembering a mentoring relationship. A foster child needs an adult who can meet weekly, talk things over, discuss the future, and compare notes about growing up.

If you feel your foster child needs such a person in his or her life, see if there is a Big Brother/Big Sister program in your community and place the child's name on the waiting list. Many communities have programs for a child to find a mentoring friend like this. It may take a few phone calls and a little patience, but the wait will be worthwhile.

You and the child and the other adult should have an understanding that the child must always be safe and all activities must be healthy. Obviously sexual activity is off-limits for such an adult-child relationship. You may not want the adult to smoke in front of the child or there may be other areas of concern. Talk directly to the adult, when the child is not with you, about these concerns. You need to consider the ultimate best interest of the child.

MUSIC AND THE FOSTER CHILD

At any age, children can learn to enjoy music. The music they enjoy may or may not be what your family likes. This is an area in which you need to be culturally aware and tolerant. Hispanic music or Israeli music or Russian music can be obtained in a large record store or in a library. Play it, learn the words, and let the whole family enjoy it together.

A foster child should always be given the opportunity to sing. It is a wonderful way to bring pleasure into life. Children who appear to be poor singers may improve with some encouragement. The church choir or the school glee club may be appropriate for an older child who can sing. Be available to help the child learn the tunes and the words or find a family member who can help.

Dance is an excellent outlet for a child's energy. There are dance classes in many community centers and children's agencies. Dance is also a way for a child to maintain his or her heritage. African Americans have dance styles quite different from those of European Americans. Encourage the foster child to participate and praise his or her skills.

Instrumental music may be more difficult. In a public school music program there may be instruments to borrow or rent. Practicing regularly may be a difficult challenge that you and the foster child cannot handle. The foster child who goes from place to place may not be able to maintain an instrument and gain skill. If he or she does want to start an instrument, try to encourage choosing one that is owned by the school and used at school. Drums, string bass, and tuba are such instruments that do not need to be bought or transported.

CULTURAL AND ETHNIC DIFFERENCES

Differences between foster children and their foster families are quite common. An African-American child may be placed in a Caucasian home, a gay teen may be placed in a heterosexual home, or a Bosnian child may be placed in an American home. The child may be concerned about these differences. A foster child faces many losses and losing ethnic ties represents an additional loss. The child may also feel inferior or inadequate because of his or her differences.

One way to help prevent problems about cultural differences is to discuss this from the beginning with the birth family. Ask about their customs and religious activities. If there is a language difference, try to make sure the child does not lose the ability to communicate with the birth family. "Juanita was in an Anglo foster home for three years and when she went home, at the age of five, she couldn't speak Spanish any more," a caseworker said.

If there are ethnic or cultural differences between your family and the foster child, find connections with similar people outside of your home. Speak highly of persons who are different from you and who are similar to your foster child. See if the school or caseworker can identify a mentor or friend who can spend an hour a week with the child. Talk to the teacher about celebrating appropriate holidays in school. Keep the child involved with events in the community that would allow her to have pride in her roots. Borrow books, tapes, videos, and magazines from the library that are appropriate for the child and her heritage. Find posters for the walls. It is especially important to have pictures of African Americans if that is the background of your foster child.

Work with your own family, your relatives, and your neighbors. Help them feel positive about this child, who comes from a different cultural background. Eliminate culturally uncomfortable words from your home, such as terms that one might use to apply to foreigners, to African Americans, or to gay persons.

When you face difficulties with a foster child, remember that you love the child and that, most of the time, she is having a good experience with your family. Talk with the child and listen to her views. Enjoy what the child can teach you about her heritage. Whenever possible, make adjustments within the home to accommodate the child's cultural needs.

RELIGION AND THE FOSTER CHILD

Probably you know the religion of the birth family, and very likely it is not the same as yours. A foster child of any age should be allowed to participate in his birth family's religion. Try to figure out a way to make religious services available on a regular basis. Speak with clergy from the child's religion and discuss the problem with him or her. Perhaps a member of the congregation could take your foster child to religious activities or perhaps you can take the child yourself.

The child may ask to participate in your family's religious life. If that is going to happen, you must discuss it with the birth parents and the caseworker. Then approach it cautiously and let the child know that he should consider returning to his own religion when going home.

What if you are not religiously active? Only about half of American families are involved in their chosen religion, although most identify themselves with a religion. If your family is not religious, give the child an opportunity to develop a religious interest. Talk to the birth parents. That may be a way for the birth parents and the foster child to get back together.

Try to learn as much as you can about the child's birth religion. As the child grows older, there may be times when he should become more involved in it. Continue to offer opportunities to participate in religious activities as the child grows older. Religion is especially important in the African-American community. The teachings are often quite practical and personal. Young people who participate in such a church will learn a special kind of strength that will be useful throughout life.

PLAY

Some experts consider children as essentially "working" when they are playing. Children may play alone or with others. Parents tend to be contented if children play quietly and if they are not interfering with the adults' activities.

Until about five years of age, children do not play very well with other children. Adults are needed to keep order. The term "parallel play" describes how several children may play in the same room but not interact with one another.

Rough-and-tumble play looks a little like fighting. This is a common type of play in four- to seven-year olds. The actions may be similar to fighting, but there is little sign of anger. There may be some unwritten rules for this type of play. It can be difficult for a foster child, who enters a new neighborhood, to understand and participate in rough-and-tumble play in the new environment.

Dramatic play is a type of play activity in which children essentially create a story. There may be costumes and props just like a real dramatic production. Again, there are often unwritten rules and customs. This type of play is also difficult for a foster child to partake in with a new set of children.

Foster parents may need to provide supervision for a young foster child who is learning to play with new friends. Allowing the interaction to take place in your house may help. You may want to interact, yourself, for a while. You also may need to keep the time periods short.

Children of any age may play alone. While playing alone, toys are not shared and activities do not involve other children. This play may be quite satisfying for a child and may be the most appropriate type of play for a foster child. Foster parents can step in and out of this type of play. Providing materials, costumes, and appropriate snacks can encourage play. There may be imaginative aspects just like with dramatic play.

If your foster child plays well alone, but not with others, try to interact with him yourself to get the child started playing with others. Teach him about sharing, listening, playing fair, and not hitting.

CLUBS, SCOUTING, AND FORMAL ACTIVITIES WITH OTHER CHILDREN

A foster parent can do a child a huge favor by starting him or her in some type of organized activity, such as scouting. The child will be able to fit into another similar group wherever he or she goes next. There may be an opportunity for success or leadership that this child does not find in a classroom. A further benefit is that there may be enough adult supervision to allow the child to attend without the presence of the foster parent, providing foster parents a chance for a trip to the grocery store or a nap.

For a child there will be an opportunity to sample various crafts, games, and group activities. The child will feel quite normal, as all of the children are working towards a similar goal. He or she will be exposed to materials and to ideas that may be new. This will broaden the child's perspectives and bring about new levels of sophistication.

Some foster children with behavior that is problematic or immature cannot spend time riding bikes and playing ball with neighborhood children. These children may do much better in a structured setting. For such a child, you may want to find several after-school activities for different days of the week. If there are costs involved, there may be special subsidies or scholarships for foster children.

SPORTS FOR THE FOSTER CHILD

Certain sports are appropriate for foster children as the child moves from home to home and back to the birth home. Try to interest the child in sports that can be played in various settings and that are not costly. Basketball, soccer, and track may be good sports for a foster child. Foster children may not be able to manage some team sports. Baseball and ice hockey may involve parents in the neighborhood and long-standing teams and relationships. Other team sports may require a lot of patience and a willingness to lose, and these features may present difficulties to the child.

A foster child may not have the talent or the competitive edge to play sports. If a child is interested in a sport, try to practice with the child regularly. If you cannot do so, try to entice a neighbor to help. Whether or not the child is in sports, play or walk with the child regularly. It will keep you both fit and give you a wonderful time to talk.

Many foster children have not learned to be good sports. A game may end up with pushing, yelling, or crying. A good coach may be able to help with this and if the child has athletic talent, it is worth trying to work through these difficulties. It is especially hard for a foster child to lose, as he often feels that life has treated him unfairly.

Your foster child would be better off finding one favorite sport and developing specific skills. If you can influence the decision, it should be a school-sponsored sport that does not require expensive equipment and financial support from home.

Use the interest in sports to discuss and implement healthy changes in diet, to discourage smoking, and to discuss safety habits. Good sportsmanship, as learned on the athletic field, will be helpful in making this child feel good about himself. And being good at a sport will bring praise and success to the child.

SAFETY ISSUES IN SIX- TO TWELVE-YEAR OLDS

Many parents now take it for granted that their children will buckle up when they get in the car. When a new foster child enters a home, he or she may not have this habit. Make sure you actually check, for a while, to see that the seat belt is fastened. Talk about using seat belts in cars that belong to other persons.

Bicycle riding is an important part of growing up. Safety is a concern when a child rides a bike, especially the risk of head injury. Make it a family rule that everyone wears a helmet when riding a bike. That way, it will be quite acceptable and there will be no arguments.

Fire has a fascination for most children, as well as adults. Make sure that lighters and matches are locked up and put up high. It is all right to teach a child to light a match under your supervision, but do not allow matches to be used in play. If a foster child has a history of fire setting or is particularly interested in fire, special precautions must be taken, such as extra supervision and extra smoke detectors.

Guns, weapons, and firearms cause nothing but tragedy and heartache in a home. If they are kept in the home, they should be locked, unloaded, and kept up high. The ammunition should not be located with the weapon.

USING LEARNING EXPERIENCES

As infants, children learn the names of things and they learn what those things can do. This learning is a result of many experiences that allow a child to explore and gather information. As a child gets older, he learns about things that he does not actually see. During the elementary school age, the child asks many, many questions as he continues to explore the world.

A foster child who comes to your house midway through childhood may need help to begin the learning process. It is important that your home be a place where people learn. It should have the materials and the quiet environment for learning, and family members should have curiosity and an interest in learning.

The foster parents should be optimistic about the child's ability to learn. Teach the child to be persistent. If he is trying to learn to ride a bike or memorize a song, encourage him to try over and over. Life is a series of challenges, and you can help the child feel good about success.

A child's failures can be as important as his successes. When a foster child does not succeed in something he has attempted, ask what happened. Have the child think about how to do it the next time and what he learned from failure. In that way, the child is almost constantly learning.

GETTING READY TO EARN A LIVING

In the elementary school years, you will not be teaching vocational skills to your foster child. However, you do need to help the child learn basic skills that will be helpful in the work world in the future. Teach him to start something on time. Encourage the child to complete a job and praise him for that.

Find small jobs for the child around the house that will be similar to those in the working world. Show him how success in this small job will lead to job readiness in the future. The child will gain self-respect by doing a job that is important to you. These should be considered contributions rather than chores. Suggest ways that a child can solve a problem, rather than solving it for the child.

Cook together and make sure he or she masters all kitchen skills that are appropriate for a child of that age. Food service careers are plentiful, and often they are easy jobs to get. The skills the child has learned at home will be important. Always teach good handwashing while working with food.

Projects around the house will be especially helpful for the child if they are done in the spirit of teamwork. If you need to carry a heavy object, have him carry one end and teach him to communicate with you as you go through doors and hallways. Good communication skills are quite helpful at a worksite.

TREATING FOSTER CHILDREN WITH RESPECT

All children may complain of lack of respect. However, this is often a major issue with a foster child, whose life has been turned upside down through no fault of his or her own. These children often feel rejected by their own family, by their friends, and by their community. They enter your home needing a lot of support. You need to encourage them and to respect them. "I felt like he was such a tough little kid, to have gotten so far on his own. I told him I really, really respected him for his self-reliance," said an older son of a foster parent.

Foster children have opinions and it may be new for them to be able to express them. Their social skills may not be very good, so help them learn to express opinions and ideas. Listen to the child and nod quietly. Do not indicate that he or she is too young to have such opinions. Think of yourself at that age sitting at a stranger's kitchen table, and respect his or her opinions.

Many children in foster care have developed a way of communicating with adults that involves complaining. "I've got a sore throat" or "Jimmy took my crayons" are comments that serve to get an adult's attention. The child needs to learn to get attention in other ways. When that kind of complaining starts, try to listen and then put it aside. Continue the conversation in a more positive way. The child may be so pleased to be listened to, that he feels better.

A child learns respect by watching others be respectful. You demonstrate respect by not interrupting family members when they are speaking. Show the child the way you respect your own children, your spouse, and your parents. Expect a reasonable amount of respect from the foster child towards you.

NUTRITION

Normally children begin to explore various foods as they get into the elementary school age. A foster child may be delayed at the "pickiness" stage of a preschooler. In that case, try to find out what the child likes, give adequate amounts of that food, and slowly introduce new foods. Praise such a child if he tries something new.

A good diet for an active child in this age group includes protein, carbohydrates, such as bread and pasta, and lots of fruits and vegetables. Fruits and vegetables can be as simple as canned peaches or as complicated as a spinach soufflé. Although it is recommended that persons eat five servings of fruits and vegetables a day, this may be hard to manage unless the foster parent is constantly monitoring the diet. Be sure to include milk.

Many children are overweight, just as many adults are. If obesity runs in the child's family, it may be hard to change. If you focus on adding fruits and vegetables to the child's diet, you may help to encourage better eating habits as those foods seem to cut down on hunger. Make sure there is a lot of physical activity. Do not consider it a defeat if the child is overweight or gains excessive weight with you. Many Americans are overweight and it is not easy to prevent this.

For all children, limit junk food. Do not buy potato chips, candy, and soda on a regular basis. These can always be picked up for a special occasion. When you feel like baking, do something with potatoes rather than cookies. Learning good nutritional habits will be helpful in bringing up a foster child who eats well.

DENTAL CARE

Normally, it is recommended that children first go to the dentist around the age of three. This is often difficult with a foster child because of the payment source. Generally three- to five-year olds do not need any fillings or other procedures. Whether or not you can find a dentist, important preventive measures should be taken.

Be sure the child knows how to brush his or her teeth. Most children are willing to brush once or twice a day, but they may not know how to do it. Get a child-sized soft toothbrush and show the child how to scrub the teeth, up and down, all around, inside and outside. Use toothpaste with fluoride. If you live where there is no fluoride in the water, talk to your doctor about fluoride supplements. Also check the child's teeth periodically. If they look all right in a preschooler, you can probably wait until school age for the dentist.

By school age, you must have the child see a dentist at least once a year. It is important to be positive about a dental visit. If you do not let on that you are afraid, the child may not even think about being fearful. Sometimes foster children are surprisingly brave about things like dental visits.

If a child comes to you and already has obvious cavities, or if the dentist recommends a lot of dental work, you may want to find a clinic where costs will not be a problem. Avoid having general anesthesia administered for dental work. Most children tolerate the mild discomfort of modern dentistry without needing to be put to sleep.

8

School

Children usually start school around the age of five, although handicapped children may start much earlier. School is an extremely important part of life for children, and success in school tends to bring success in later life.

For foster children, school may be especially challenging for several reasons, including frequent moves from one school to another. Studies show that foster children are often behind in their academic level when compared with others their age. Behavior in school may be a problem for such a child. School attendance and performance in school often improves during the time that a child is in foster care.

Foster parents, who may have these children for brief periods, should consider ways to work together with the school and teacher to help the child find some success, develop good study habits, and learn as much as possible of the required material. The school and teacher should represent part of the team, working together for the benefit of the child.

MAKING FRIENDS IN A NEW SCHOOL

Children who feel a little different often have problems in school. Foster children are always the "new kid in the class." There are certain things you can do to help a foster child fit in. Make sure that he or she is dressed appropriately, make sure the child is clean and neat and that the hairstyle is similar to that of the other children.

It is always easier to enter a new situation with a friend. Try to find a child in the neighborhood who can help the foster child for the first few days of school. Recess and lunchtime are particularly difficult for new children. After a few days of school, the teacher may be able to suggest a friend for the foster child. Call that child's mother and try to arrange a trip together to a skating rink or some other appropriate activity.

In general, you should offer to pick up other children for activities or have them over to your house. You will get a chance to see how your foster child interacts with other children. Try to help the foster child learn to get along with others, to be a good listener, and to share when appropriate. If the visit does not go well, wait until the friend is gone and then ask the foster child, "What did you learn?"

After a few weeks in a new school, talk to the teacher about the child's adjustment with the other children in the classroom. Ask him or her if there are ways to make this child feel more comfortable and fit in better. Then go over this information with the child. It is very important that this child learn to adjust to new situations, as his life will probably continue to involve frequent changes.

GETTING STARTED IN A NEW SCHOOL

Some children find new situations frightening. Others, and this includes many foster children, are not flustered by change. Make sure the child knows your name, phone number, and address. Be sure the school has that information, and if you are not home for the first few days, make arrangements with the school for a way to reach you.

The school will place this child in a classroom and then will evaluate that placement over the first few weeks. In terms of schoolwork, the child may be delayed and he may have been placed in a more advanced program than he can handle. If this happens, the school may recommend a change in classroom or may suggest ways you can help. Foster parents should work quite closely with the school for the first few weeks. Tell the teacher that you will be available to help whenever he or she calls you. If it appears that you will have to work with this child at home, make sure you understand the instructions from the teacher.

If the child has any problems that are health-related, speak to the school nurse. Prescriptions are usually necessary for medication given at school. If the child occasionally wets herself, send along a change of clothing. If the child needs to be reminded to go to the bathroom, tell the teacher.

Behavior problems and mental health problems may be something you know little about. If you have heard details of this child's misbehavior, you may want to keep them to yourself for a while. If there are issues of safety for the school, such as firesetting or extreme aggression, inform the school authorities. Otherwise, let the child's behavior develop on its own.

FEELING GOOD ABOUT SCHOOL

Foster children are sometimes teased within a school, and that may make the child quite uncomfortable. Talk to the child about trying to ignore some of it, but if it seems to be excessive, you or the child should talk to the teacher. The teacher may or may not be aware that a child is feeling uncomfortable, but he or she should be able to change the situation for the better.

Another problem these children may have in school is that their academic skills are often poor. Many have had such a difficult time of life that learning did not occur. "I brought two sisters and a brother into my home, aged seven, eleven, and twelve. None of them could read or write," said a foster mother. If the child is in the lowest reading group, or goes out for special help, or has to repeat a grade, the foster child may feel quite uncomfortable. Be optimistic about any setbacks and tell the child that he will be moved into the regular program when he catches up.

School may be very difficult for a foster child. He may need to use extreme effort in order to behave well and in order to learn. Each part of the day, he may be confronted with the need for skills he lacks. Be sure the child understands that you are sympathetic. Give praise for his efforts and encourage him to rest a bit when arriving home.

Foster children often do not feel that school is important for them. In their previous life, there was little evidence that academic success was meaningful. Such a child may not have seen adults who were successful. You will need to demonstrate the significance of learning for most foster children.

POOR PERFORMANCE IN SCHOOL

There are often serious school problems with these children for obvious and not-so-obvious reasons. If the child is having trouble in school, be sure you have visited the child's doctor and discussed the problem. Make sure the child does not have lead poisoning, anemia, or thyroid problems. See that hearing and vision are normal. These are the most common physical reasons for getting behind in school.

If the child continues to do poorly in school, have the school arrange for a psychological evaluation. It may be time to consider medication for hyperactivity or for depression. The school psychologist and the child's doctor can help you and the child. Be sure to involve the caseworker in this process.

If school performance does not improve, talk to the teacher, counselor, school social worker, or principal. Ask to have a special conference to talk about your foster child. It will give you a chance to speak to several people at once. Ask to have the birth parents and the caseworker present. All of these adults will focus attention on the child's problems and suggestions from such a meeting may be quite helpful.

Make sure that everyone at the school knows that you love this child and you care how he does at school. Do not accuse them of doing a bad job, but do encourage them to change their ways if you think they are being too harsh or that they are not handling the child well. Encourage the teacher and others at the school to praise this child whenever he does well. Foster children are more likely to respond to love and positive attention than they are to punishment and criticism. Let the school know that.

GETTING EXTRA ACADEMIC HELP

If the child is not keeping up in school, there may be helpful resources. Ask if he would benefit from any kind of therapy, such as speech therapy or occupational therapy. Ask if a special teacher for part of the day would help or an aide in the classroom. If you ask pleasantly about these things, you may be surprised that the school will be cooperative. You should all feel like part of a team, working together for the child. Use your good behavior, as an attentive parent, to help encourage school personnel to show an interest in the child.

There may be help for the child outside of the school as well. People may be available to tutor a child after school through agencies or libraries. Read articles in the newspaper or make phone calls to see what is available. If the cost is high, there may be special financial arrangements for this child because of his status in foster care.

You or a family member may be quite a help to a foster child who is struggling in school. Sit with the child and give him special attention for about fifteen minutes every day. Spend some of that time with formal schoolwork and some just challenging his mind.

LEARNING DISABILITIES

Learning disability means a disorder of language that makes learning difficult. This term is not used if the learning difficulty is caused by a vision problem, a hearing problem, or by mental retardation. Experts say that about fifteen percent of children are learning disabled, and studies show that it is more common in foster children than in other children.

Children with learning disabilities look and act normal. However, when you ask questions, such a child may show difficulty in answering. He may not understand the question, may have difficulty thinking through the problem, or may not be able to put an answer into words. These are problems that prevent the child from performing well in school.

The advantage of making a diagnosis of learning disability is that the child will get special help. He will be given extra time and extra resources in situations that might otherwise be quite stressful. Teachers are quite good at helping these children learn special skills to work around their problems. A child who cannot write may learn to express himself out loud by taking an oral test. Sometimes a child with serious problems will do better in a special classroom where there are fewer students and all of the students have similar problems.

SPECIAL EDUCATION

For a school-aged child, if there are learning problems, special education may be appropriate. Such classrooms have fewer children and more adults than a regular classroom. Children placed in these classrooms usually have learning problems, behavior problems, or both. The books and other materials may be different from those used by children in regular classrooms and are usually easier. Teachers in special education are experts at dealing with learning and behavior problems. Additionally, teacher's aides usually work with the teachers, and schools often have social workers, speech therapists, and occupational therapists available for children in special education.

If your foster child is in a regular classroom and you think the child needs special education, you may have to advocate for the child. Talk with the teacher or principal about your concern. Special education classrooms may not be located in the neighborhood school, and transportation may be separate from the bus used for neighborhood children.

If a child does well in a special classroom and is to be moved back to a regular classroom, there are ways to make that change gradually. Some schools "mainstream" such children by putting them part-time in a regular class and part-time in special education.

If a child in special education changes schools or districts, he or she can usually be placed in a similar classroom. Be sure to keep a copy of school records to send on with the child.

THE FOSTER CHILD WHO IS BRIGHT

Even though foster children may have been through bad times, you may discover that the child is really bright and has the potential to do well in school. If the child is doing well at the present time, continue to encourage him, providing plenty of opportunities for learning and praising his successes.

In other cases, a child who seems bright may not be performing well in the classroom. You may know that the child is intelligent from the results of psychological testing or you may just suspect that he or she is bright by observing the child in your home. Most adults feel that any child should be working up to his or her capacity. If the child seems to have the potential to do better in school than he is doing, seek help. The teacher may understand why the child is not doing well and know how to improve his performance. Ask if tutoring is available for the child. Special programs for talented children are available in museums, libraries, and colleges. Try to access such programs. Try extra hard to advocate for this child while he or she is in your care.

TEACHING STUDY SKILLS

Foster children often do not have good study skills. One mother said, "I finally sent her to her room to study and when I went in, she had torn her book into shreds." Professionals often say that parents should not be involved with teaching study skills and with homework; however, with a foster child you may need to be involved.

At the beginning, if the child has homework to do, ask to see it. Ask the child if she understands the assignment. Suggest a quiet study area, such as the kitchen, and make sure the television is turned off. Expect studying time to be short in the beginning, so have the child do the more important work first. If she has questions, try to help without giving away the answer the teacher is seeking. Keep an eye on the child and when she is finished, ask her to read parts of the work back.

As time goes by, help the child learn to organize the work. Make sure notebooks are neat and she makes a list of assignments. Consider preparing a box with the child's name on it for storing school supplies and anything needed for school the next day. You may want the child to produce a chart for each subject and each day. She can then check the box for work completed. This allows you to monitor the work and praise her successes. Teach the child to proofread her own work for accuracy.

Talk to the child about schoolwork once a day, perhaps while preparing supper. Ask about tests and assignments done in class. Ask about successes and praise them. Ask about things that did not go well and then ask, "What did you learn?"

After a few weeks, ask the teacher how the foster child is doing. If homework assignments and other work are satisfactory, step aside and allow the child to progress without your help. If things are not going well, you may need to continue to monitor study time and help with study skills for some time.

A LEARNING ATMOSPHERE AT HOME

Your foster child should find your home a pleasant place to learn. Learning involves a lot more than just schoolwork. Your home should have books in it, both for you and for the child. There should be books to read aloud to the child and books at the child's reading level. Go the library with the child frequently. Make sure she has a library card of her own that can be used after leaving your house.

Play word games while driving in the car with the child. Tell the child some of your experiences, then listen while she shares her own experiences with you. Ask questions and show your interest. When asking the child to do things at home, make sure you have her attention by saying something like, "Ready?" Then give short instructions with only two or three steps. The instructions should sound more like suggestions than orders. Before the child starts the project, ask if she understands. This allows the child to succeed and allows you to praise her for her success.

Try to coordinate activities with school projects. If the class is doing a special project on autumn, go out and collect colored leaves, coat them with wax, and have the child take them to school. Have craft material in your house. Allow learning to be noisy and active within your own home. Listen to a child's wildest ideas and occasionally accept one. Use anything that happens through the day as a "teachable moment." Ask the child if she understands what happened, add to her ideas, and then talk about what has been learned.

Make activities in the kitchen learning experiences for the child. Encourage her to cook a few things well. Ideally, she should be able to make all parts of one meal, and this special meal should be prepared on a regular basis, with assistance from you if necessary. Try to encourage the child by cleaning up together after she cooks. Praise the food that she makes.

HELPING A CHILD LEARN TO WRITE

Everyone needs to learn to write, and this is a skill that can be encouraged by many activities at home. As soon as the foster child is able to hold a crayon, begin to teach him to write his name. The alphabet can be sung before most children can recite it. Soon after learning the alphabet, the child should begin to write it. As soon as the child can write a little, have him sign cards for members of his biological and foster families. The child can make or buy simple cards for holidays and birthdays. Make a list of important dates so he can plan the cards ahead.

As the child begins to develop reading skills, have him write little stories for you. The stories can use easy words, like dog and cat. Have the child illustrate the stories and read them back to you. When the foster child is old enough to write more complex things, have him make grocery lists for you, and write notes to delivery people and menus for the family. His writing skills will grow and, with it, his ability to communicate. The child's grades in school can be expected to improve due to your efforts with him at home.

THE FOSTER PARENT AND THE SCHOOL

As a foster parent, you are a professional parent, and, ideally, the school should treat you as one. You need to act in a manner appropriate to that role. Dress well when you visit the school. Carry a notebook to write things down. Smile and praise the teacher and staff who work with your child.

Everyone needs to be recognized for the good things he or she does, and teachers often feel unappreciated by parents.

Try to be as helpful as possible to the teacher. Do not send the child to school if she is sick. If there has been a crisis and you can predict trouble at school, send a message to the teacher. If possible, be around at the end of the day occasionally to pick up the foster child and talk to the teacher. Consider being a room mother. Go to all PTA meetings. Offer to bake or bring in healthful snacks. If you are serious about your role as a professional mother, the child will get treated a little bit better at school.

If you wish to make suggestions to the teacher, sit down with him or her alone. Use good listening skills, briefly describe what is bothering you, and then listen to see if he or she suggests a solution. Do not gossip to other mothers about the teacher and do not complain to the principal until you have tried to handle any problems directly with the teacher.

Get to know the office secretary and the aides in the child's classroom. Sometimes these are the persons who will help your child. Always praise the teacher to the staff and principal. You cannot do any harm with such praise and it may benefit you and the child. If your child is having problems, you may want to set up a system of communicating daily with the teacher, by note, about academics or about behavior.

ADVICE FROM TEACHERS REGARDING FOSTER CHILDREN

Teachers admit that foster children are often problematic in their classes. Most schools are fairly homogeneous, with similar children in a classroom. Foster children tend to come from a more impoverished background. They are often at a different academic level, their behavior is often different, and they often have had a history of abuse and difficulty.

As the teacher may be worried that this child will cause extra trouble, he or she would appreciate your sending the child to school healthy and well rested, with homework done and school supplies organized. Teachers want to know if there are any special safety or behavioral issues concerning the foster child. If the child has been aggressive, has demonstrated unusual sexual behavior, or has set fires, the teacher may need to make special preparations. Teachers also want to know if there are medical concerns like asthma or epilepsy. They do not, however, need to be told personal aspects of the child's past experiences.

Teachers appreciate involvement from a foster parent, although they may not wish to have you in the classroom for long periods of time. Teachers welcome a foster mother who drops in occasionally to read a story to the whole class. Teachers are sometimes uneasy about the motivation of foster parents. They may suspect that you are "just in it for the money." They will gain respect toward foster parents as you and they work together for the benefit of the child.

DROPPING OUT OF SCHOOL

In many states, school is optional for children over the age of sixteen. That means that children can drop out at that age and the court will not make them return to school. Dropping out of school, however, generally has very serious consequences. If a foster child drops out of school, he or she probably will not be able to remain in foster care. The child will have to return to the biological family, move in with friends, or become homeless. It would be quite unusual for a seventeen- or eighteen-year-old young person to become self-supporting.

Do anything you can, as a foster parent, to keep a foster child in school. Talk to the guidance counselor and see if any kind of extra academic help would be useful. A tutor or a mentor at school might make a big difference. Sometimes a change in schools or moving the youngster into a vocational school or some other alternative school will be appropriate. Try to make this move as quickly as possible once a child over sixteen has significant absences.

While trying to keep the child in school, you should nevertheless begin to work on work-readiness and housekeeping skills. Help the child fill out necessary forms and applications so that the community services will be available after the child leaves foster care.

9

Adolescents and Teenagers

Some foster parents specialize in teenagers. They find that these older children bring very special challenges and rewards. As children grow older, they begin to understand more about themselves and the world around them. Because of this understanding, discipline is handled a little differently. If teens are treated like children, they tend to rebel. Teenagers need to talk things through with foster parents, and in these discussions there should be some level of agreement.

Issues of independence normally surface during the adolescent years. Teenagers struggle between strong ties to adults and the need to take care of themselves. With foster children, these issues of independence involve biological parents, foster parents, caseworkers, and judges. Independence is an appropriate goal for most foster teenagers.

HOW TEENAGERS THINK

When children reach the teenage years, they develop a more adult style of thinking and they have a broader understanding of the world around them. At the same time that a child is developing a broader view, the teenager also seems to focus on himself. A teen tends to be sensitive and easily embarrassed, feeling that everyone is looking at him and being critical. This is particularly difficult for a foster child, who may truly get negative attention from others.

During the teenage years, language skills grow and a personal style develops. This style may be cynical and negative, or it may be upbeat and light-hearted. Teens begin to think in terms of possibilities, either realistic possibilities or fantasies about the future. A teenager may tell you about plans that he has developed and be interested in your reaction.

As opposed to younger children, teens can often see all sides of an issue. That feature of teenage thinking leads to a tendency to turn everything upside down. Teenagers are able to argue persistently and can sometimes take either side of an argument. Teens tend to rebel against adult authority. They rebel against parents, foster parents, teachers, and every other authority. Teens may rebel about relatively unimportant areas of daily life, such as hairstyle and clothing choices. On the other hand, they may rebel about important issues that involve safety and health.

ADOLESCENT STRESSES

Many teens feel quite stressed by everyday life. They often feel that people are not treating them fairly, that life is hard, and that they are not liked or loved. So there are natural stresses for all teenagers, even those who are not in foster care.

A foster child may discover things about himself or the biological family that make him quite uncomfortable. There may be poverty or drug abuse in the biological family. He may feel that the problems in the biological family will make his or her own life extremely difficult.

Lack of financial resources can be quite stressful for a foster teen. The child may wish for possessions and for money. Also, as other teens begin planning for college and career training, this child may feel that there will be no financial support for him once the teenage years have ended.

If your foster child has been in special education or has been considered retarded or delayed, that may cause discomfort when the child becomes an adolescent. Older children may be very unhappy about being identified as handicapped.

Sexuality causes difficulty for many foster children. If they are developing an interest in the opposite sex, they may not be able to attract partners. If their development is leading to an interest in same-sex partners, they may have a very difficult time.

If a young person is going to become violent or is going to harm other people, this will begin in adolescence. Teenagers with these behaviors are often worried and feel that their lives are out of control.

MORAL DEVELOPMENT

Moral development tends to take place in the early teenage years. This consists of knowing what is right and what is wrong, how to be kind, and when to obey. Most foster parents expect some immaturity in foster teens, as the children struggle to understand what has happened to them and how they are going to fit into the adult world. Many foster children have spent some time in institutions and this lifestyle may have caused delays in moral development. Employees of institutions may try to encourage good values, but the closeness of the other troubled children may result in some difficulties.

In helping a child learn good moral attitudes, discuss universal principles like the Golden Rule and the Ten Commandments. If you or the child feel uncomfortable using religious language, talk about what is "good for all." Society expects adults to make decisions that are good for all whenever possible. Ask the foster child questions like, "What would you do if a friend asked you to shoplift?" Then help the child work out an answer. Moral values are best taught by example. If a problem occurs in your home or community that provides such an example, discuss it with the foster child. Try to tell the child about your own decisions and the important moral values that you used to help make those decisions.

Children need to develop sensitivity and kindness to others, including the disabled and those with racial differences. It may take a lot of in-depth conversation to convince a foster child that these values are important. If you are successful in teaching sensitivity towards others, this may be one of your most important accomplishments.

RULES

With younger children, your rules must be accepted and obeyed. A teenage foster child needs actually to agree that the rules are necessary. In the teenage years a person gradually becomes an adult. Adults set their own rules, so this is a transition period between childhood and being an adult.

You may have a few household rules that cannot be broken. Those involve safety and health. You may prohibit smoking in the house or you may not allow fighting. Other rules, such as curfew time and homework time, may meet with enormous resistance. Research shows that setting rules is the commonest area of conflict between parents and teens. At the same time, studies indicate that a child not subject to rules will have a lot of trouble.

Adolescence is not a time for parents to be permissive. It is a time where rules will be discussed and argued about. Parents will give up some childhood rules and will concentrate on important safety and health issues. They will need to help teenagers establish their own rules for taking into the outside world and for taking into the adult world.

FRIENDS AND HOW THEY INFLUENCE FOSTER TEENS

Friends can be very important to a child, especially a foster child. They may provide a source of information and they may be supportive. Peer pressure can be helpful, as friends encourage a child to learn new skills.

Your foster child may tell you a lot about her friends. Children tell you more if they think you are listening and interested. Try to keep track of the friends' names and ask about them often. Ask the child about alcohol, drugs, and sex as part of these discussions. If you suspect that your foster child's friends are a bad influence, talk to adults who might know these children. Ask the school about them. There are generally adults who can advise you on whether or not you should be concerned.

If you determine that there is a problem, taking strong action may be difficult. You sometimes cannot stop a friendship when you want to, but you may have some luck talking the foster child into your way of thinking. Talk to the birth parents and to the caseworker. "I went to court with Towanna when the kids were all picked up for shoplifting," said a foster father. "I had heard that there was a lot of drinking going on with those kids. I asked the judge to speak to her and he did. He told her that she had an opportunity to clean up her life now, and get away from those kids."

WORKING PART-TIME

If part-time work is part of the plan that you and the agency have for this child, help the child proceed with getting a job. For a foster child, such part-time work may be part of career planning, as he or she will need to be self-supporting as a young adult. It is important to plan ahead about the money that will be earned. Make sure you, the child, and the caseworker have a plan for how the money will be spent or saved.

Schoolwork may suffer, if part-time work requires significant time and energy. Make sure that everyone agrees on the motivation for working. Consider urging the child to work during school vacations, rather than during the school year. See if there is a job around the neighborhood or with a friend at the beginning.

Starting a job usually requires filling out forms. The school usually does some of the paperwork, and the employer should know the relevant laws, such as rules about children working late at night or long hours.

If you are helping a child find work, think about his or her strengths. Try to steer the youngster toward an area where you can expect success. Advise him or her on various aspects of working, such as starting on time and dressing appropriately. Being successful in the work world is very helpful in building self-esteem.

PREVENTING DELINQUENCY

Unfortunately many foster children have parents who are incarcerated or who have a history of criminal behavior. Although this does not mean that the tendency will necessarily be inherited, it usually means that the family members do not handle stress and poverty well.

If you have had this child for a while, you may have done everything you could to prevent illegal behavior. You have talked about drugs and stealing. You have tried to help him understand what is right and what is wrong. Studies indicate that a child who has good bonds with a parent or with another adult is likely to stay out of trouble. If you and your family are not providing a mentor, you may want to find such an adult who can guide the child.

If your foster child has been accused of shoplifting or property damage, sit down and talk with him. Foster children often offer excuses indicating that they could not help what they did. Tell the child you do not want to hear excuses. Do not let him think that this behavior was acceptable. Talk with the child at length. Talk it through and go over the situation. Discuss methods of making decisions and methods of managing anger. How should the child react the next time he is tempted to commit such an offense?

WANTING A CHANGE IN PLACEMENT

Many foster teens go through periods of wanting to move out. Even teenagers in intact families may wish to leave home. So the first thing for foster parents to remember is that this happens to many parents, from time to time. Such foster parents should not feel that they have failed. Sometimes they have done a good job of parenting and the child is expressing a real need for change. It is important for the child to talk to the caseworker and to his or her birth parents. Everyone needs to know what the options are for this child.

In many cases, efforts should be made to keep the child in your home. Foster children have had at least one family breakdown and another one may be quite harmful. Everyone needs to talk this over and decide if your rules need to be changed, if the child's behavior needs to change, or if there are other ways to keep the child with you.

For a foster teen, there are several alternatives to staying in your home. Returning to the birth home might be an option. Perhaps the child will fit in with his family better than when he was younger or perhaps the biological parents have made some changes. If abuse was a factor, older children are much less likely to be abused than younger children.

The second possibility is that an older teen might move into a group home. Some communities have group homes in which teens live in a supervised setting. Independence is a goal and the child is taught to take care of himself or herself before being discharged. Perhaps you, as the foster parent, would continue to be a resource for this child.

Of course, a move to another foster home might be arranged. There may have been differences in culture or religion or language that could be eliminated with a move. A kinship home that was not available earlier might be found, allowing this child to live with his or her own relatives.

RUNNING AWAY

It can be expected that many foster teens will run away from the foster home. In some cases, the child has run away before and nothing you can do will totally prevent it. Some child care experts point out that a child who runs away is seeking independence. He or she may decide to live with a neighbor or a friend for a few days.

Your caseworker may have indicated rules for you to follow should the child run away. Very likely you will need to call the caseworker. Try not to call the police for the first day or two. Instead, try to locate the child by calling friends' parents and asking if they have seen the child. If you locate the child, send a message, such as, "Tell her that I love her and she is welcome back whenever she is ready."

If you cannot locate the child or cannot get any assurance that all is well, you and the caseworker may decide to call the police. However, the situation is likely to escalate if the police find the child and bring her back. The child will be angry and the police may be demanding. Very likely, a child who is brought back by the police will not be able to stay with you.

When a child returns from a runaway experience, give her a quick hug and tell her you are glad she is back. Send the child for a shower or a nap, and tell her that you will discuss it later. When everyone is calm, sit down and discuss what happened. The child will expect an appropriate consequence, such as grounding or loss of privileges. Provide a reasonable consequence that you can enforce. The child has tested your resolve by running away and you need to prove that you can handle this.

If running away occurs several times, there may need to be changes. School may be inappropriate, the child may need a part-time job, or placement may need to change. This may be the time for the child to go back to the birth family. Talk everything over with the child, the birth parents, the caseworker, and the school authorities.

FOSTER CHILDREN EXPLORING THEIR ROOTS

Almost always there are cultural differences between the foster child and the foster family. These may include differences in language, race, religion, or education. Older foster teens may want to explore their cultural heritage or they may want to reconnect with the birth family. That may be an appropriate time to look for other relatives to get involved with this child. It may also be the time to encourage the child to learn his original language, attend religious services in his birth religion, and so on.

If a foster child has not seen the biological family for many years, getting back together may be quite distressing. The birth family may be involved in drugs or other illegal activities. Also, the birth family may have had more children and your foster child may feel he or she has been replaced. If you suspect that such a late reunion will be disturbing, talk with the caseworker before encouraging visits.

Sometimes a return to the biological family goes fairly smoothly for a teenaged foster child. This child may be old enough to overlook the bad treatment he experienced before and sympathize now with the biological family. "Tim lived with me from the age of seven to eighteen. When he was twenty-two, he brought his birth mother to meet me. I had never met her before. They seemed pretty happy together," said a former foster mother.

GANGS

Gangs serve as an alternative to families for some adolescents who are not getting satisfaction at school or at home. A child needs to have some successes and, unfortunately, he may look for success in the world of gangs. You can help prevent gang involvement by encouraging a foster child to find areas where he can succeed. It is important for foster parents not to set goals that are too high. Praise all accomplishments, even if they are small. If a foster child feels a lack of encouragement, he may turn to gangs, where the child hopes to "get some respect."

Ask the school about gang activity. Learn about some of the habits and styles that will let you know if your foster child is getting involved. Do everything you can to prevent him from joining a gang. There are no good aspects to gangs. They are dangerous, and children may be injured, killed, or go to prison.

As soon as you have an idea that this problem is beginning, sit down and talk with the child and the caseworker. You might want to make a deal that if the child stays out of a gang, he can stay in your home. Tell the child that he cannot live in your home and be a gang member. Gangs tend to have a very violent style and encourage their members to become violent. Talk to your foster child about jail and the criminal system. Tell him that if he is caught in criminal activity, he will be moved out of the foster care system and into the juvenile justice system.

If your caseworker is not helpful, find someone who can help. This is a specialized area. It takes an adult who understands the gang system to deal with these children.

USE OF TOBACCO

Many children start smoking at the age of thirteen or fourteen. If family members smoke, a child is more likely to start smoking. In your case, you may also have to deal with tobacco use in the biological family. Although most adults agree that smoking is a bad habit, it continues to be taken up by young teenagers, who consider it a sign of sophistication. Make sure your foster children know that you do not want them to smoke. Talk about the risk of cancer and heart disease for those who smoke. Be sure they know that you care and that you will be quite disappointed if they begin to smoke.

If the child's school allows smoking, either by the students or by teachers, you should advocate for change. There should be no smoking in school or on school grounds, and teachers should not smoke in school.

Remember that it is illegal, in most states, for children to buy cigarettes. Never buy cigarettes for your foster child and never ask your foster child to buy cigarettes for you. Tobacco is considered a "gateway drug," meaning that children who smoke are more likely to use other drugs. If your foster child smokes elsewhere, insist that he or she not smoke in your house or your car.

DRUG ABUSE

The drug habit most common among impoverished young children is glue sniffing or inhaling other substances. The substances inhaled are readily available and inexpensive. The side effects can be severe. Nausea, headache, seizures, and sudden death can occur from these activities. If a child is spending lots of time alone, if the material is available to him, and if he has a rash around his nose, then you should consider the possibility of an inhaled drug.

Cigarette smoking is another way children begin abusing substances, afterwards possibly also using alcohol. Cigarettes and alcoholic beverages are available at reasonable prices and are easy to steal. Smoking and alcohol use do not usually result in a child going to jail; they do, however, cause mental confusion and a decrease in judgment.

Marijuana, or pot, is so common that many young persons assume it is not an illegal drug. It is widely available, inexpensive, and gives a pleasurable sensation. It is, however, illegal. The foster child should know that the use of illegal substances would get him into serious problems quickly because he is already involved with the court system.

Drug activities may be attractive to teenaged foster children because of the opportunity to make money. Most foster children are unhappy with their poverty, so their involvement with cocaine and other drugs often begins as a way to earn money. Even if they eventually start using drugs themselves, they are usually looking for an escape, or a way out of a bad situation. They may use drugs to feel better, rather then taking drugs to feel good.

You should talk to your foster child about all of these problems. You do not want him to end up in jail. "I remember when Travis was a freshman in college. We were so proud of him. Then he got arrested for having sold drugs in the high school. That was considered a federal crime," said a caseworker.

ALCOHOL

Foster children may have come from a home where alcohol caused problems. A woman who drinks alcohol while pregnant risks having a child with behavior problems and low intelligence. This is called "fetal alcohol syndrome" and is common in foster children. There is no specific treatment.

Many foster children have witnessed terrible problems due to alcohol. Their own parents may have been confused under the influence of alcohol and have been abusive as a result. Alcohol may be one of the main reasons that these children are in foster care. Nevertheless, that often does not stop them from trying it. They may consider the use of alcohol as a natural part of growing up. Organizations and self-help groups for children of alcoholics may be appropriate for a teen whose own parents have alcohol problems. Such groups are very caring and may help the child stay away from alcohol use.

Whether or not you drink alcohol, you should be strongly opposed to your foster child drinking at all. If your foster teen experiments with alcohol and you know about it, make sure that the child understands how you feel. Do not serve alcohol to anyone under the age of twenty-one in your household. Do not allow a foster child to drink your alcohol. Do not buy alcohol for your foster child. Do not let your child drink and drive.

In the later stages of alcohol use, your foster teen may become addicted. In that case, try to motivate the child to enter rehabilitation. Most communities have alcohol abuse agencies where you or your foster teen can get advice.

EATING DISORDERS

Anorexia nervosa and bulimia are relatively unusual in foster children. These eating problems tend to occur in young women who come from affluent families. The problem usually begins in the mid-teens and can last for a lifetime. Persons with anorexia nervosa demonstrated weight loss, starvation, and an obsessive increase in exercise. Bulimia involves binge eating and vomiting after eating; it usually does not result in weight loss. In both cases, these young women have an abnormal perception of fatness and are quite concerned about their appearance.

Sexual abuse in the past may be a factor, although that is not always the case. These eating disorders are diagnosed and treated by doctors and psychologists, usually working as a team. If you have a child with such an eating disorder, you will be asked to monitor the amount of food eaten. The child may need consistent encouragement to eat appropriate amounts of food and maintain an appropriate body weight. Sometimes hospitalization is required. These eating disorders tend to persist into the early adult years, with symptoms worsening at times of stress.

DATING

Interest in the opposite sex is a natural part of growing up. Dating presents new pleasures and new problems for foster children. A foster child may expect a girlfriend or boyfriend to supply what is missing in his or her life. At the same time, the foster child's social skills may be inadequate to attract or keep a partner.

The foster child may have unreasonable expectations of success in dating. As a foster parent, you can encourage discussion about dating behavior. You may be able to present problems for the child to discuss, such as, "What would you do if your date gets mad at you?" If you have older children who can advise the foster child, bring it up at the dinner table.

Foster children have had many losses, so the loss of a girlfriend or boyfriend may be especially stressful for them. A broken-hearted foster teen may be quite vocal and unhappy. Expect to spend extra time with the child if a relationship ends. Be as reassuring as you can. Watch closely for signs of serious depression or for hints of suicidal thoughts. Get professional help if the child is having significant problems.

With a foster child, as with any child, you need to discuss abstinence and safe sex. Be sure the child knows what your values are. Your views may be more or less strict than those of the child's birth parents. Let the child know what you expect and help the child develop acceptable behavior.

The first few times your foster child dates, you should stay up for the child. Keep a light on and be there to greet him or her. It is a time for talking and it is vital that the child knows that you were concerned and you cared whether or not the evening went well.

BIRTH CONTROL AND SAFE SEX FOR FOSTER DAUGHTERS

If you wait for your foster daughter to tell you she is sexually active, you may wait too long. Very often children begin having sex without thinking of the consequences and also without telling their families. For a foster child there are special reasons for this to happen, as they do not usually have a strong relationship with a parental figure. If you suspect that your foster daughter may be thinking about sexual activity, start talking about it. Make sure she has information, and if you feel she needs more, get advice from professionals. Talk about the potential for date rape, the possibility of getting infections, about HIV/AIDS, and about pregnancy. If you think you have told her everything, tell her again. She will be listening to you each time, even if she looks like she is not.

Tell her that you or the caseworker or her birth mother will take her to a family planning clinic if she wishes to go. Also, let her know that, in most states, she can go to such a clinic by herself. Advise her of that and make sure she knows where it is and how to get there. It is acceptable if you tell her that your first choice for her is abstinence. You may not want her to have sex, but it does not make much sense to leave the conversation there. Too many young girls become pregnant for foster parents to ignore the possibility.

If your foster daughter is willing to use a method of birth control, the injections are probably best. A shot of Depo-Provera lasts for three months. If she will let you help her, write down her appointment for the next shot and make sure she goes. If she chooses birth control pills, offer to help her remember to take them. Other methods of birth control are too chancy for most adolescents to use. Birth control injections and pills will not protect against infection. A young woman must to insist that the boy use a condom.

Unfortunately, many adolescents seem to want to have a baby. Consequently, birth control methods may be unattractive to those young women. This is particularly common for foster children as they often are looking for someone to love. This is an issue to talk over with the child and the caseworker.

SEXUALITY AND FOSTER SONS

When a foster son begins to date, there should be conversations about dating. Do not expect a foster child, on his own, to understand how to handle himself. Talk about each step of dating, from making the phone call to saying good night. Foster parents are often quite comfortable with this type of conversation, as they have discussed it with each teenage foster son who has come to them.

Your foster son needs to know how to act when he is out with a young woman. Tell him about dating etiquette, such as walking on the outside, opening doors, and holding her coat. Do not expect him to have already noticed this type of behavior.

Be very direct when you talk to the child about sex. Tell him, if you want to, that he should remain abstinent. However, you must also talk about issues of sexuality that may be important for him. All sexual activity must be consensual; in other words, the girl must be agreeable to having sex with him. Then, every time he does have sexual relations, he must use a condom. Tell him the condom is for his protection, to prevent infections, and also to prevent pregnancy. Make sure that he knows about getting girls pregnant. If sex with a young woman results in pregnancy, he will be responsible for helping raise the child. Try to discourage any fantasies he may have about being able to do so.

You cannot discourage dating and sexuality and you should not. Be open about your relationships and those around you. Let your foster son know that he has many years to be together with the woman of his dreams and that he should wait a few years to make a commitment.

PREGNANCY IN FOSTER DAUGHTERS

Girls can get pregnant as soon as they start their periods—even before. Most adults feel that teenage girls should not get pregnant. Nevertheless, there are many factors that lead to teen pregnancy. Being a foster child makes this concern even greater. Obviously, if pregnancy has occurred, the young couple has not used birth control. They may not have planned ahead, not wanted to use a condom, or they may have been overcome by romance.

Many girls actually want a baby. Adults often assume that a young teen would not want to be burdened with a child, but often the youngsters really want to be parents. Their fantasy of having a baby and showing it off and loving it makes it seem reasonable to them. When asked how she is going to support the child, a girl may say, "I'm going to marry Alec and he'll quit school and get a job and we'll get a house." This may seem impossible to you, but quite reasonable to her.

All of these issues are more common in foster children. They are often forgetful, often romantic, and often have fantasies. An additional reason for pregnancy is that a foster daughter may realize that pregnancy will get her out of her present placement. It may allow her to go back to her birth mother or to be independent.

If your foster daughter becomes pregnant, make sure she knows all her options. She can have an abortion, she can give the baby up for adoption, and she can keep the baby. Most family planning clinics can discuss the options and help plan an abortion, if she decides to do that.

FOSTER DAUGHTERS HAVING BABIES

Many foster parents would feel that pregnancy in a foster daughter is a real defeat. However, once the baby is on the way and abortion is no longer an option, your thinking must be turned around. The new child has to be welcomed and the new mother has to know as much as possible about raising a child.

If the girl is older, she might actually settle with the baby's father in an independent situation. Another possibility is that she and the baby might go back to her birth home. The environment of her relatives, who will help with the child, may be good for the baby. Perhaps the whole situation that resulted in your foster child's removal from her parents has changed.

If the pregnant teen stays in foster care and wants to keep her baby, the child will probably enter the foster system. Then, if you wish, the mother and her child might stay in your home, or they might go to a group home with supervision. The caseworker will be involved in the planning process. The young mother does have some control over the infant's placement.

Whatever the outcome, early in the pregnancy there will probably be several weeks of making arrangements. During that time, make sure the pregnant teen goes to a prenatal clinic even if she's going to deliver elsewhere. Make sure she gets vitamins and takes them. Keep an eye on her diet.

Try to be nonjudgmental about the pregnancy. Your relatives should also be as kind as possible. This girl is going to be a young mother and she needs everyone's support. Teach her all that you know about babies. If she is leaving you, tell her that you will always love her and that you will want to visit back and forth before and after the baby is born.

HOMOSEXUALITY

First remember that some children, usually between the ages of eight and twelve, will have some problems with "gender identification." Such children are not sure if they are boys or girls. The foster child has so much trouble with self-identification anyway, that this may just add to the confusion for him or her. In those early phases of developing sexual identity, try to be flexible. The child may just need more information about looking and acting feminine or masculine. He or she may need a little help with clothing, voice quality, and mannerisms.

As children enter their teenage years, they may begin to show signs of bisexuality or homosexuality. Again, remember that this may be an experimental stage. It may go away in time and you should be careful not to perpetuate the identity by commenting on it, teasing the child about it, or insisting upon changes. Some adults clearly are homosexual and many of those persons found their altered sexual identity as teens. Your foster teenager may be in this situation, feeling strongly that he or she is gay. You should be very, very accepting.

There are two reasons to be accepting. One is that homosexuality, in many cases, seems to be beyond the control of individuals. They cannot change, even if they might wish to. The other reason is the possibility of depression, low self-esteem, and suicide. Foster children should be considered somewhat fragile anyway, and this kind of lifestyle feature may be too much for the child to handle.

There are counselors who can be helpful, but you might have to look for one. Likewise, you might have to seek out support groups for teens who are gay. There is a whole world that this child may end up moving into and you may need to learn about this world.

If your child is male and appears to be gay, you will need to talk about safe sex and AIDS. It may be easier to talk about this than you think. The child is probably dealing with the same concerns and can use your help.

For some reason, many persons become angry in the presence of gay people or around people suspected to be gay. They become so uncomfortable that they actually abuse gay people by calling them names or physically attacking them. For that reason, many experts recommend that a young person not "come out," that is, not admit that he or she is gay until after high school.

BECOMING INDEPENDENT

Nonfoster children generally stay involved with their parents until they reach their mid-twenties. In most states, foster care ends at the age of eighteen, and many children drift out of foster care even before that age. There are several options for a foster child who "ages out" of the foster care system. A child may go into an independent situation, may return to the biological family, may live with friends, or may become homeless. In many cases, the youngster ends up in an unsafe environment. Often there is not enough to eat, and the child must steal to survive.

Some foster parents have said that their most important job is to teach common sense. Foster children need to be taught to ask other people for help. They need to learn to manage money, to take care of a household, and to cope with public transportation. For foster children, there is a special need to gain these skills, as there will not be a parent to help them after the age of eighteen.

You can help a young person learn to fill out application forms. The child may need to apply for work, for college, for welfare, for nutritional supplements, and many other things. Unfortunately, many foster children do not have the reading and writing skills to manage these forms. Work with the child to know what basic clothes are needed. Help the child shop at discount stores for clothing and other supplies. Teach the foster child to buy groceries and to prepare simple meals. Make sure the child knows how to do laundry.

10

Helping Foster Children Learn New Behavior

When a child has been removed from home, he or she has the opportunity to make many changes in the area of behavior. Foster parents can be an important influence in helping foster children make these changes successfully. It is important to remember that the nature of childhood is growth and change. As children grow up, their behavior should become more mature and they should become more independent. Ideally, when a person comes to the end of childhood, the young adult is able to live within a family and able to earn an income.

Foster children generally have not been able to move smoothly through the normal stages of childhood. They may have been held back at an earlier stage and immature behavior has persisted. In some cases, development has gone in unusual directions and behavior is abnormal. Immature and abnormal behavior may prevent a foster child from reaching independence as an adult.

HELPING ALL CHILDREN GROW UP SUCCESSFULLY

Most foster parents have raised their own biological children and so they already have some experience. Raising children requires a special set of skills, and biological parents use a variety of resources to learn these skills. They consult with family members, they read books on child care, and then they see if their methods work out.

Normally, young babies are able to get parents' attention easily, either by crying or by smiling and waving their hands. Parents respond to attention-seeking behavior in a baby by picking the infant up, cuddling the child, and sometimes offering food. The infant learns, early in life, that parents are available and helpful.

When babies become toddlers, parents begin to teach them how to make decisions. Parents tell children that eating before dinner will ruin their appetite or going too fast on a tricycle will make them tip over. A parent may also add consequences, telling a child that she cannot watch television if she continues to tease her brother.

As children reach school age, the parents are not always available for immediate guidance. Parents talk things over with their children before sending them away from home. They explain about school behavior and getting along with other people. Children generally follow their parents' guidelines when they are away from home.

Parents also provide a model for good behavior for children. Parents wear seatbelts in the car, for instance, and therefore the children learn that it is appropriate to wear seatbelts. Being a good role model is an important part of parenting.

Families have certain rules regarding verbal and physical behavior. Adolescence is a time when normal children begin to test the family rules. Teenagers try their own hairstyles, have music preferences, and choose their hours of sleeping and waking. Most families realize that a certain amount of conflict is to be expected as teenagers grow into adults.

For most families, when a child has successfully reached adulthood, he or she will have received all the education that is necessary, will have a job, will have moved out of the house, and will have started to establish a new household.

HOW FOSTER CHILDREN HAVE GROWN UP

For many foster children, normal methods of parenting have not occurred. Your foster child's biological mother may have been young, may not have had advice from others, and may have been inattentive to her child. She may not have had knowledge of ways to handle children and she may not have known how to get the information that she needed.

The crying or smiling baby may not have gotten picked up, hugged, or fed. From the very beginning, disturbing patterns may have been set, where the child's smiles were ignored or where the child was not handled in an appropriate way. In the toddler years, when children are beginning to learn to make decisions, the foster child may not have had an attentive parent. Possible consequences of actions may not have been described before an activity, and, afterward, there may have been no one to discuss the consequences with the child.

The stage of introducing a child to outsiders, which normally begins in school-aged children, may not have occurred. Such a child, who cannot get along easily with others, has an increased likelihood of difficulties in foster care and throughout life.

Most foster children have not had good role models in their lives. Parents have not acted wisely. Many of these children have seen violence and abuse, poverty and neglect. The adults around these children have provided poor examples for their children. Rules were not clear in these households, where tempers flared and resources were scarce. Consequently, if the child became an adolescent in that home, the normal rebellion against household rules may have led to enormous confusion.

THEORIES OF CHILD DEVELOPMENT

There have been many theories about the way that children develop. The early theories of child development, sometimes called "psychoanalytic theories," amounted to lists of stages that children were thought to pass through before they reached maturity. Each stage had to be passed through smoothly in order for a child to grow up without problems. Any child who had been mistreated would, according to these theories, require years of intense professional help in order to thrive.

As a reaction to the psychoanalytic theories, "behavioral theories" were developed next. These theories suggest that a child's behavior is influenced by the way caregivers react. Certain behaviors in babies are reinforced by parents smiling and praising the child. Other behaviors decrease because caregivers ignore them or show disapproval. According to these theories, if parents react wisely to a child's behavior, good behavior will develop.

A third set of theories implied that parents could teach a child to behave well. It was proposed that children actually learn a lot by what they are taught. This is the "cognitive perspective." These theories say that there is usually a step between the cause of a behavior and the behavior itself. This step is the process whereby a child decides what to do, and if the child does not think logically, abnormal behaviors will occur.

Looking at these theories of child development, one might be discouraged about the possibility that any foster child can do well. However, a fourth set of theories involves resiliency. It appears that certain children do well despite an upbringing that might have seemed quite unacceptable. These children, who succeed despite adversity, are considered resilient.

The suggestions in this chapter for changing a child's behavior are based on a mixture of these theories. Foster parents tend to follow a common-sense approach to raising children, and in most cases that approach works quite well. Foster parents, pediatricians, and caseworkers have offered many suggestions for raising foster children effectively, and these suggestions are included.

RESILIENCY AND FOSTER CHILDREN

Psychologists are now using the term "resiliency," which literally means bouncing back, or thriving, even when there are difficulties. Resiliency is a good thing and there are ways to recognize persons who are resilient. Your challenge is to change a foster child, to help that child become more resilient.

In order to be resilient, a child needs people, resources, and opportunities. The child's environment should include a significant adult, or parent, who consistently guides the child and serves as a role model. Resources should include food, clothing, books, and items such as toys and bicycles. In addition, the child should have opportunities to learn and to succeed. You, as a foster parent, can provide people, resources, and opportunities for a foster child. You and your spouse are role models. You provide food and clothing. Your family and the community provide opportunities.

In addition to having supportive people, resources, and opportunities, certain types of children seem to be particularly resilient. To be resilient a child should be cheerful and optimistic about the future, do well in school, have problem-solving skills, and get along well with others. You cannot make a person optimistic and cheerful by just telling him to be that way. However, as you model cheerfulness for the child and reward a cheerful child with praise, there will be a gradual change. There are many ways to help a child succeed in school and to learn problem-solving skills. Getting along with others may not come easily to foster children, but you can help.

One aspect of resiliency research that is good to remember is that, although these factors suggest that a child will do well in the end, the child may not look very resilient when he is with you. One former foster mother said, "She left us at sixteen and went into a psychiatric facility. I thought she would never live independently. She was so messed up! And then last week, six years after she left us, she called us from across the country. She's going to college and she wanted us to know how much she appreciated everything we had done for her."

ATTACHMENT

Attachment, or bonding, is something that usually occurs in the first few months of a child's life. Attachment is a loving, nurturing relationship that forms between parent and child. If a child is placed in a foster home as a newborn baby, attachment can proceed in a normal way between foster parent and infant. In the case of an older child coming into a foster home, he or she may have missed the bonding experience because of poor parenting. It now appears that if a child misses the bonding experience early in life, attachment can occur later in childhood if a loving caregiver is involved. However, attachment may take longer, in such a child, than the attachment that naturally occurs immediately after birth.

While in foster care, some children do not seem to bond well with foster parents, and this can lead to difficulties. An "unbonded" child may act remote and unresponsive. Such a child can present problems for foster parents, especially as foster parents tend to be affectionate and nurturing. Such parents can become quite discouraged if a child does not respond to them and does not laugh or smile.

Many foster parents are concerned about attachment problems. They feel that such "unbonded" children are difficult to care for. They suggest that a single or unmarried foster parent should not take such a child, and that there is a need for extra help in terms of relatives or respite care. They believe that such a child tends to have an underlying feeling of hopelessness, a feeling that is hard to change.

An "unattached" child needs to be handled with consistent loving care. Parents should have reasonable expectations for responsiveness. This may not be a child who will hug you a lot. The child will do best with structure and with many opportunities to learn to accept love and attention. Children with attachment problems may seem unaware of what is going on and they may not develop good safety skills. They may wander away from home or into the street.

More serious disturbance seems to occur in some children who lack attachment, including defiance and aggressiveness. These children may not respond to the usual approaches to discipline. "Time-out" may not be effective, because the child may not mind being away from other persons. One foster parent described a "quick scolding" as the only way to communicate with such a child when the child was misbehaving.

Another aspect of attachment is the feelings that a foster parent may develop toward the foster child. This type of attachment is healthy and causes no harm to the child. However, some adults fear that they may become "overly attached" to a child. Some foster parents feel that it is not safe to get too attached. They fear that caseworkers will notice that and move the child elsewhere. They also fear that their own feelings of desolation when a child leaves will be overwhelming.

DECISION MAKING AND PROBLEM SOLVING

Many foster children do not make wise decisions. They have grown up in a tumultuous environment where there was no time to think out all the consequences of an action. In their struggle to manage, they often took the easiest way out of a problem. They also tended to approach a problem the same way others in their family did.

You may feel you have to go back to early stages of decision making with a foster child. You need to help these children understand the natural consequences of their actions, even simple actions that you might expect children of their age to already understand. Concepts such as "Yelling in the house makes Mom unhappy" or "Helping set the table makes Mom happy" may need to be pointed out over and over. Try to use situations where the consequences are predictable. You may feel that you are teaching the child common sense, but that is appropriate if he never learned common sense.

If a child continues to make quick and inappropriate decisions that lead to trouble, help him learn some technique for thinking things through. Use a device, such as the "Stop and Think" approach. This is a five-step program used whenever there is a problem to face. First, tell the child to stop and think about the problem. Then, ask him to consider different things he could do. Third, have the child decide which to do. Have him do it. Afterward, ask him how it worked out.

Help the child work through the first four steps when likely situations arise around the house. If two children want the same toy, have the foster child think of different ways to proceed. Afterward, remember to ask how it worked out and if another choice might have been better.

An older child often has problems that occur outside of the home, and the child should be prepared to use the skills you have taught him. Be sure to take advantage of issues that arise at home and take the child through the process, then encourage him to use the same process when away from home.

Some foster parents become very good at teaching problem solving. They may use a "Stop and Think" approach or a "red light/green light" approach. One former foster child said, "I can always hear Joan's voice telling me to stop and think. It still helps me to figure things out."

DISCIPLINE

Discipline is the way a parent encourages a child to have acceptable behavior. It is also the way parents deal with a child who has broken a rule or is misbehaving. Psychologists feel that it is best for a child to be taught good behavior by rewarding that behavior whenever it occurs. That begins when parents reward a smiling baby by hugging and cooing, and it continues throughout childhood by making sure that there are rewards for a child who behaves well. Teaching a child to cooperate with others in this manner allows the child to learn the advantages of behaving well.

Foster parents arrange their homes so that there is room to play and they set reasonable rules. When a foster child participates in family activities or plays quietly, the foster parents reward the child with praise. Sometimes a foster child may not feel the need to follow your wishes. The child may say, "Why should I obey you? It never helped me, when I was with my folks. I just got treated bad, no matter what I did." Do not allow that kind of reasoning to go unchallenged. Tell the child he is in a new place, with new adults who will always be reasonable. As time goes by and you praise the child when he is cooperating, he will learn that it is nice to be appreciated.

Cooperation is encouraged by pointing out logical reasons for that cooperation. As an example, if you tell the child, "If you set the table, we can eat sooner," he or she can understand the reasons for cooperation. Another way to encourage good behavior is redirection. If a foster child starts to do something that is annoying or harmful, try to distract him. "When Shawn started to run around the house and act crazy, I used to put on my sneakers and go out and throw a ball back and forth with him. When he got older, I could send him out on his bike."

Discipline should include helping the child understand the consequences of actions. Sometimes those consequences will happen naturally and you simply need to point them out. A foster parent can say, "If you're late for school, you'll get a bad grade on the test."

TIME-OUT AND OTHER CONSEQUENCES OF MISBEHAVIOR

Sometimes foster parents need to create consequences when a child is breaking rules or misbehaving. This is similar to punishment, but differs in that it is fair and reasonable and does not involve anything physical, like hitting the child. Consequences for bad behavior may include a lecture from you. Try not to sound angry and try to be alone with the child. Point out firmly that the child is breaking rules. Remind him of the need for such rules. In this discussion you may want to develop a consequence for the child's actions if he does it again. This should be a logical consequence. If the child comes into the kitchen with dirty feet, he should be expected to mop the kitchen floor, but not to mop the whole house.

For younger children, if firm words have not helped, the next step may be "time-out." Time-out means that, since the child is not following your directions, you will take the child out of activities long enough to get cooperation. This involves putting the child in a special spot, like the bottom stairstep or a quiet corner of the living room. Tell the child he must settle down. After settling, the child must stay in time-out for a period of time. Following that quiet time, the child needs to express, in some appropriate way, that he will change the offending behavior. Then he can go back into the action.

Time-out is appropriate between the ages of two and ten. The recommended time-out period is usually one minute per year of age. Try not to seem angry or frustrated when putting a child into time-out, as it is not supposed to be punishment. It is supposed to be putting the child in a quiet and safe place until he settles down.

Some foster parents point out that a child who has not yet formed a relationship with a foster parent may accept time-out a little too easily. He may not mind it at all and that defeats the purpose. Time-out begins to work when you and the child have a relationship, so that he is sorry that you are not interacting during that period.

For older children, your consequences usually involve suspending privileges. Whenever possible, this should be matched to the misbehavior. The period should be short, and then you should stick with it. "I couldn't stand the arguments over the computer games, so I said no one could play them for twenty-four hours. It sure was a quiet twenty-four hours," said one mother.

Physical punishment is problematic in foster care. You may have spanked your own children, but it is seldom appropriate for foster children. If you are handling an especially difficult child, you may get involved in restraining a child who is overwrought. You should not do this unless you have worked out the details with the caseworker.

HELPING FOSTER CHILDREN WITH TEMPER TANTRUMS

For children who live with their own parents, tantrums may occur around the age of two. Toddlers use tantrums as a way to get what they want and as a way to get attention. Parents tell toddlers that tantrums are not acceptable, and they help their children to learn ways to deal with anger, like taking a few deep breaths or going to the car until the angry feeling passes.

Often, a foster child has not passed smoothly through the tantrum period. She continues to yell and scream to try to get her way and also to get attention. If your foster child is having tantrums and the child is quite young, use the same approach you did with your own child. Try to avoid situations where tantrums occur. If a tantrum starts, ignore it if possible or remove a child if necessary. Never give in to a child who is having a tantrum. For most young foster children tantrums go away naturally.

HELPING A FOSTER CHILD CONTROL ANGER

Temper tantrums in young children usually occur when children want something they cannot have. Older children may become angry for the same reason, but their anger is often more focused on other persons. Anger is often part of a foster child's personality and that is somewhat understandable. However, anger must be kept under control, and foster parents can be quite helpful in teaching this.

If your foster child has problems handling his or her anger, talk about it at a time when you are both calm. Discuss ways that angry outbursts can ruin friendships and stand in the way of success in school. Suggest ways to avoid yelling and shouting. The child could take some deep breaths or count to ten. Some children learn to take pride in walking away from situations that make them angry.

Foster parents can teach a phrase like, "Think first, act afterwards." The foster parent says this phrase out loud when the child appears to be getting angry. After a few times, it is whispered. If the method is successful, the child learns to say the same thing to herself. This is called "self talk," and it can be quite effective if a child is motivated.

You may want to develop logical consequences for an older child who loses control. Discuss your rules with the caseworker and make sure the caseworker is in agreement. Any rules and consequences should be discussed with relatives, teachers, and biological parents.

Anger management is just as important for the foster parent as for the foster child. These children often seem to cause feelings of anger in adults around them. When you feel yourself becoming irritated, use whatever methods of self-control you have tried to teach your foster children. Use your own self-talk. Your angry feelings will be apparent to the child, and as she watches you, she will learn how you manage your own anger. If you resolve the situation in a healthy way, both of you will have gained by the experience.

COPING WITH AGGRESSIVE BEHAVIOR

A child who is angry may be tempted to hit or harm someone, and this is called aggression. Your foster child may attack another child directly if that child has made him angry. The foster child may also feel the need to hit back if he is hit first. Although fighting is not rare among adolescent boys, it should be discouraged. Be careful that your own family members do not encourage this type of fighting. Telling a boy to "act like a man" or "stand up for himself" is not appropriate in today's society.

If an adult has made a child angry, very likely the child will not be aggressive toward the adult. If that child chooses to become aggressive, he will probably hit or harm someone his own size. So whenever hitting or fighting starts, you need to talk things through to try to find the true cause.

Foster children may have grown up in an environment where there is a lot of hitting. The child's father may have beaten the child's mother. The foster child himself may have been beaten. For such a child, the tendency towards aggressive behavior will have to be unlearned. When you reprimand this child, the child may respond with, "Why shouldn't I hit him? I got hit all the time in the past." You need to explain that hitting is not the way to get ahead in the world, and you probably will have to repeat this many times.

Studies indicate that watching television and playing computer games encourage aggressive behavior. You cannot entirely prevent these activities, but keep in mind that the influence can cause problems, especially for a foster child who may already have aggressive tendencies.

If your foster child continues to fight and be quite aggressive, you will need professional guidance. Try to find a counselor who can meet with the child on a regular basis. Speak to the caseworker and make sure a plan is developed to attempt to change this child's behavior.

IMPULSIVENESS

Foster children often act impulsively, or without thinking. Although serious forms of impulsiveness require professional help, mild forms can be handled by most foster parents. Acting quickly in a thoughtless manner usually results from stresses in a child's biological home or in previous foster placements.

An impulsive child may ask you questions, then repeat the same questions over and over. Most of the time, he does not seem to listen well to your answer. The child may seem rude as he jumps from thought to thought. Also, this child may move about quite actively, so that he may damage clothing and items in your home.

Probably this child has had problems in school because of restlessness. One thing that may help is to get the child involved in a physical activity, such as martial arts. Karate and other martial arts programs actually focus on slowing down one's thoughts and on ways to relax. This can be quite helpful to such a child. Also, evenings will be calmer if the child has been active after school with sports or some other physical program.

If the child has not been involved with the biological family, that may be causing stress. Try to set up visits with his biological parents. You may be surprised to see the child settle down if he knows he will see his parents regularly.

Go to school and meet with the teacher. Talk about things you are doing with the child at home and find out what methods are being used at school. Work at home with this child on homework. Sit with him for fifteen minutes each day, working a little and just talking a little. An impulsive child may show significant improvement if a foster parent works with him to help him slow down. However, sometimes professional help is needed, and medication may also be helpful.

HELPING FOSTER CHILDREN MAKE FRIENDS

Normally, children progress from having friends selected for them and meeting with them under adult supervision, such as toddlers in a play group, to being able to choose friends and interact with them away from home. Friends provide companionship, mental stimulation, and physical activity. Maintaining a friendship requires certain social skills. One of the features of a resilient child is the ability to make friends and keep them. As a foster parent, you can be a big help to a child by teaching him ways to make and to keep friends.

Whatever age your foster child is, you will want to provide opportunities for friendship. Consider preselecting the friends and supervising their activities at the beginning. This will allow you to keep both child and friend comfortable and to help your foster child learn new social skills. Your supervision may include providing craft materials, toys, and snacks.

Talk to your foster child before the children get together. Tell him that they will have to play together in an appropriate way. If they get into mischief, you will be unhappy. Then, after the visit, let the foster child talk to you about the experience. Many foster children are ashamed of not having a family of their own. "Jimmy bragged about his own family, all the time," a foster child may say. Let your foster child talk this problem out and offer a few suggestions.

Over the time a child is with you, help him learn the importance of giving to others. Have the child make birthday cards for his friends, perhaps help a friend on a paper route. Teach him generally to take an interest in the friend. Ask the foster child questions that will stimulate his interest in the other child, such as, "What books does your friend like to read?"

Older foster children know that they may be moved to another home and, consequently, may lose the friends they have made. Let the child talk to you about that as well. Suggest ways to keep in touch with friends if such a separation occurs. Talk about your own friends and how they have been important in your life. The foster child will meet these people, watch you interact, and absorb everything you and the friends say. When you argue with a friend, tell the child that this sometimes happens, but it does not destroy a friendship.

A resilient child has what psychologists call a "prosocial" attitude. This means that the child takes an interest in others, is appropriately sympathetic with others, and tries to please others. As you help a child develop these traits, you will have made a difference in his future.

SEXUAL BEHAVIOR

In most families, sexual activity is quite a private matter. Adults generally do not talk to children about their own sexuality. Most parents provide education about sex by speaking with their children, from time to time, about behavior that is appropriate. In most families, there is very little nudity, and there is very little sexually explicit talk.

Your foster child may have grown up in a family where sexual activity occurred in the open, people went about undressed much of the time, and there was sexual talk. Sex may have been used to earn money, as in prostitution, or to gain drugs or favors. The child may have learned to talk about sex in ways that your family finds offensive.

In the most abnormal families, sex may have occurred between household members and your foster child. This may have been forced or the child may have accepted it. In any case, sexual contact between children and adults is illegal and potentially harmful to the child. As time goes by, the child may tell you details of life in the biological home that make you uncomfortable. Your foster child may have been exposed to sexual behavior that was extremely damaging, both mentally and physically. Speak to the caseworker about your concerns.

In terms of the child's own sexual behavior in your home, it is important to tell the child what your limits are. A foster child may enter your home and demonstrate sexual behavior that is abnormally open and flirtatious for the age of the child. Encourage the child not to act in a seductive manner around family members or strangers. Also, make sure your family members do not respond in a sexual way to the foster child.

There should not be a rule against masturbation, as this is now considered normal. However, masturbation should only occur in the privacy of a child's room, with the door closed.

As a foster child grows older, the child's sexual development and hormone production will result in natural sexuality. As you would with any adolescent child, keep an eye on his or her behavior. Feel free to continue to tell the child that there should be no sexual activity, but also inform the child of appropriate family planning clinics. Discuss problems that can result from unprotected sexual intercourse, such as diseases and pregnancy.

READING TO CHILDREN TO IMPROVE BEHAVIOR

Reading to a child provides entertainment, is calming, and also can introduce new types of behavior. Children often understand a story and remember the moral of the story better than when you just speak to them about the same topic.

For young children, find a story that gets a point across, then read it in a dramatic way so the child really pays attention. If you are concerned about poor performance in school, read "The Little Engine that Could." If you read several books at bedtime, save that one until the end. During the day, refer back to it. You may hear the child saying, "I think I can, I think I can," and you will have encouraged him in a good thought process.

A trip to the library provides free books and also is an outing that is easy to arrange. Children tend to behave well in libraries. A librarian may be a friendly adult for a child to relate to. Make sure the child gets a library card that he can take when leaving your care.

Older children may find books that help them figure out how to manage various aspects of their lives. Ask the librarian to help if the child is interested in a particular topic. If you are familiar with the book, talk to the child about the content. After the child reads the book, ask if it was helpful.

Reading may help a child learn new behavior, but reading itself is also a behavior. When a child is able to sit quietly, turning the pages of a book, that child is taking time to think things over. When the child goes back to his original home or goes to another foster home, he will be able to produce his library card and again take up the habit of reading for pleasure that you have helped develop.

TELLING THE TRUTH

A foster child often arrives at your home without a good sense of what is the truth and what is not. Consequently, she may tell untruths that are rather fanciful. In many cases, the child is looking for love and attention, but her fantasies may cause unnecessary trouble.

Foster children often have strange tales about their life before they came to you. Many of these children truly have had difficult times and their stories can be horrifying. However, foster children sometimes tell you stories that they wish were true or stories they think will entertain you. Like any other unpleasant behavior of childhood, dishonesty may become a habit if it results in attention. Try not to overreact to things these children tell you, even though you suspect the children are not being truthful. Just let it pass, and at a time when a child is truthful, be a little more lavish with your attention.

Rather than confronting a foster child and accusing him of lying, try to put down ground rules that will prevent lying. Make sure the child knows that some behaviors, such as shoplifting or using drugs, are absolutely unacceptable.

If you have a rule against lying, make sure you do not get caught in "little white lies." This can be quite disturbing to a child who is trying to cooperate with the rules of your home. Encourage the child to be as honest and truthful as possible and praise him when that honesty might have been difficult.

11

Seriously Abnormal Behavior

Unfortunately, many foster children have seriously abnormal behavior. Some of this behavior is due to poor parenting and difficult family situations. In other cases, the cause of abnormal behavior may be genetic. If the child has been in multiple foster homes, that also increases the risk of abnormal behavior.

If your foster child's unusual behavior has persisted for several months, if it is a problem almost everywhere, and if it interferes with the child's normal activities, then you should seek professional help. Start with the caseworker and if more help is needed, try to find a psychologist or social worker to give you and the child some guidance.

Any plan that is developed should be discussed with the child, the caseworker, the teacher, and the biological family. It is very difficult to make behavioral changes and it is very important that everyone uses the same approaches.

HYPERACTIVITY THAT IS MILD TO MODERATE

Toddlers and young children are often very active. Be realistic about expectations for a child's level of activity. Normal preschoolers are full of energy, and it is hard for many parents to keep up with them. If a foster child seems hyperactive when he first comes to you, wait a while before taking action. Keep the child as busy as possible. He may be overly active because he is bored or scared or lonely. Provide as much attention as you can, and look for quiet activities that he likes.

When a two- to eight-year-old foster child seems overly active, it is recommended that you encourage quiet behavior and ignore overly active behavior. Make sure the child is safe, but try not to look or sound annoyed. Make it a habit to sit with the child a few times a day, reading a story or singing a song. Have your other children spend brief moments with him in quiet activities. Praise him when he sits still and pays attention.

If an eight- to twelve-year old seems hyperactive, talk to the teacher about his behavior. You may find that the child is not overly active at school. The child might be doing well at school and the effort to sit still leaves him too tired to behave well at home. Such a child might benefit from a snack and a rest after getting home.

If a child continues to seem extremely restless and hyperactive at home and at school, see the child's doctor or clinic. Ask to have the child checked for thyroid problems, lead poisoning, and anemia. Make sure he is not taking a medication that might cause hyperactivity. Ask the doctor about allergy or intolerance to foods, such as sugar or milk, or to other substances.

If the problem lasts for more than a few weeks, consider making an appointment with a psychologist or social worker. Such a professional may help you set up a treatment plan for the child. The plan should include ways to help the child improve his behavior, both at home and at school.

Medication may be quite helpful. It should be considered a trial at the beginning. A two-week trial is long enough to know if it is helping. If it is not helping, you may need to try a different dose or a different medication. The medication may cause poor appetite or weight loss. If that is a problem, try to rearrange pill times and meal times to increase the appetite. Whenever medication is used, supervise the child while taking it and store it up high and under lock and key.

No matter how challenged you may be by an overly active child, continue to show your love for the child. Be as patient as possible. Remember that the child is not behaving this way just to make you angry. Seasoned foster parents tend to take this sort of behavior calmly. "He'll outgrow it when he gets a little older," said a foster mother.

HYPERACTIVITY THAT IS MODERATE TO SEVERE

Some children have hyperactivity that is severe, lasts several months, and occurs in various settings. This is sometimes called attention deficit hyperactivity disorder (or ADHD), and it is particularly common in children who have come from difficult home environments and who have had many stresses in their lives. A child with ADHD is restless and fidgety, wanders about aimlessly, and has trouble concentrating. These children often seem unable to control their impulsiveness, even when they try.

Some health problems common to foster children can cause ADHD, such as anemia and lead poisoning. Identification and treatment of these problems will be helpful. Poor parenting from biological parents, plus frequent changes in foster homes, may have made the behavior worse. Frequent changes of teachers and classrooms may have led to an inability to settle down in school.

A child may come to you who already has the diagnosis of ADHD and is taking medication. The medications are safe, but the side effects may be troublesome. Most medications used for hyperactivity have to be taken frequently, and they may cause lack of appetite and weight loss. Usually the drugs act quickly, within an hour after they are given. Older children may resist taking medication that must be given at school.

Other than medication, successful treatment of hyperactivity has been hard to identify. No single approach to a hyperactive child can bring about a cure. However, foster parents may find ways to help a child learn to calm himself. For a younger child, praising good behavior and ignoring overly active behavior is the best approach. Time-out can be tried, but the time frame may need to be quite short. For older children, physical activity may be helpful, either in the form of sports or a part-time job.

As a foster child gains self-respect, the need to be constantly in motion may diminish. An older child with ADHD who is motivated to change may be able to learn ways to slow down. He may learn to repeat a phrase, or take a deep breath, or go for a short walk in order to calm himself.

ANXIOUSNESS AND FEARFULNESS

In many cases, anxieties are minor disturbances of childhood. It is common to be afraid of the dark or anxious about the first day of school. There are a few specific types of fears and anxieties that are particular problems for foster children.

Foster children may be quite nervous about future separations, either separation from you or from other persons who have become important in their lives. That is a natural problem for foster children, but most children who worry about separations can continue to function and enjoy life, despite the anxiousness. For a few children, separation anxiety becomes quite disabling.

Children with separation problems are generally not treated with medication. As a foster parent, you should consider the various ways you can help the child become brave and strong. Help him learn how to make new friends, enter new situations, and meet new adults. You cannot prevent future separations in his life, so encourage independence.

School phobia is another problem common to foster children. Often there is a combination of fear of leaving home and worrying about school itself. Such a child may refuse to go to school. In young children there may be clinginess and crying. With older children there may be truancy, skipping school, and lying about attendance.

School phobia and school refusal should be handled together with the teacher and caseworker. Different approaches are recommended for different age children. However, the adults and the child need to agree on a plan to return to regular attendance at school, after which you will have to make sure that everyone follows the plan.

"Post-traumatic stress disorder" is a term used for behavior that results from abuse. It also may be a result of an automobile accident or some other type of trauma. In foster children, it may result from disturbing events relating to the child's removal from home. Such a child may be sad, angry, have sleep problems, and have feelings of hopelessness. Children often blame themselves for the traumatic events that have happened to them. A similar disorder may occur with an adult who fought in a war and came back somewhat disturbed.

Post-traumatic stress syndrome is present in many foster children to a certain extent. Usually foster parents handle these children well. Fear of further trauma is one reason for rules about not spanking foster children. Such children need love and consistency. They need to be taught ways to take care of themselves in the future.

DEPRESSION THAT IS MILD TO MODERATE

When a foster child is unhappy or mildly depressed, there are often logical reasons. Try to help the child understand what is troubling him. If you can determine a cause for this unhappiness, you may be able to help with a solution. Do not be surprised if the child misses his biological parents, even though they have not treated him well in the past. Certain indications can reassure you that depression is not severe. If the child is sleeping and eating normally and if he has some periods of cheerfulness, this is not severe depression.

As you talk with the child about his concerns, you may find that you cannot offer any solutions. In that case, encourage the child to be strong and brave. Help him understand how he handled adversity in the past and praise the child for that. Most foster children have survived significant bad times, and they should be proud of their coping skills.

When a younger child is mildly depressed, professionals recommend that parents try to provide a loving environment and assume that the child will recover his or her good spirits. An older child will be able to benefit more by discussions about ways to cope with adversity. At any age, a child may respond well to physical activity, shopping trips, and visits with friends. The caseworker or social worker may be helpful if your foster child gets discouraged or depressed. If the child is not seeing his biological parents on a regular basis, consider trying to get visits started.

DEPRESSION THAT IS MODERATE TO SEVERE

Serious depression usually causes sadness and the sadness is present all of the time. It may be accompanied by sleeplessness and poor appetite.

There may be complaints of headaches or stomachaches. There may be talk of suicide. Sometimes depression in young children causes restlessness or aggressiveness. In teenagers, there may be increased sleeping, rather than sleeplessness.

Serious depression interferes with a child's daily activities and also interferes with relationships with friends and family. The child may refuse to go to school. If you feel that your foster child is seriously depressed, try to arrange for the professional help of a psychologist or psychiatrist. A professional will interview the child and talk to you and the school. If a diagnosis of depression is made, a special treatment plan may be developed.

The first step in such a plan is to try to break through the child's gloominess. Insist that he go to school and try to get him involved in activities. Try to convince the child to take an interest in others. A second approach is to plan a regular session with an adult who will be helpful. "We set up with my dad that Brian would go over there every Tuesday after supper. My dad likes to play catch with him and after it gets too dark, they go in and eat pretzels and talk. Brian really likes time alone with my dad," said a foster mother.

If problems with the birth family seem to be a concern for your foster child, talk to the caseworker. See if the child has misunderstood any aspects of his family's problems. Remind him that his biological parents love him and are doing the best they can. If regular visits have not occurred, see if they can be restarted.

If approaches such as these do not help, the professionals may want to try medication. Antidepressants are relatively safe, and you will see an effect within two weeks. Make sure you monitor the child as he takes the medication and see that it is swallowed. Keep the medication, and all medications, locked and out of reach of young children.

Depressed children may have certain ways of thinking. They tend to repeat phrases like "I am stupid" and "The world is stupid." Professionals will recognize these automatic thoughts and try to stop the child from repeating them over and over. The therapist may ask you to help the child understand these automatic thoughts and learn new ways of thinking.

Be very positive with this child even if that is difficult. Remind him of your love. Smile a lot and praise his efforts to cheer up. Even if the child does improve, depression is likely to return. If the child is on medication, try to keep him on it for several months. Lastly, if depression is severe, it is important to keep a child safe. Whether or not the child has talked about suicide, make sure no weapons are available and try not to leave him alone.

SUICIDE

In the most extreme cases, suicide can result from depression and the hopelessness of depression. The child may not tell you how bad he or she is feeling, but there may be hints. He may say, "Everyone would be better off without me," or "I won't be around much longer." If you hear such hints, immediately stop and talk to the child.

If you are worried about suicide ask the child, "Are you thinking of killing yourself?" If the child indicates that he is thinking about it, ask, "How would you do it?" and "When?" Take the suicide threat very seriously, if there is such a plan. If a child threatens suicide, call for help. There are certain things you can do while waiting for help to arrive. If a child is considering suicide, he is actually trying to make up his mind. Put yourself on the side to stay alive. Use the child's name when you are talking to him and tell him you want him to stay alive. Do not leave the child alone.

Do not take possible suicide lightly. If the child is thinking about it, you cannot ignore it. Do not dare the child to go ahead with it. Do not belittle the child. Do not act sarcastic. If there are specific problems in the child's life, talk about options. Try some ways to pull the child back into life. Tell the child you need him to take care of the pets, to continue his job, or that you want to take him to that rock concert you have planned. Tell the child you love him and you want him to stay alive.

Though suicide may be part of an episode of depression, it may also occur "out of the blue" or over a relatively minor problem. Suicide may occur after an adolescent couple breaks up or when a child gets bad news about school or home. It also may occur as a result of homosexual feelings of the child. Be aware of these possibilities when there are troubles in a foster child's life.

Do not delay, if you become worried. Children who consider suicide may act quickly. A trip to the emergency room may save the child's life. The child may need a day or two in the hospital. He may or may not end up returning to your home.

Treatment for a suicidal person involves close supervision, help with working out the problems of life, and medication to treat the depression. If a suicidal child is sent back home to you on medication, make certain he actually takes it. Taking the medication may keep the child alive. Supervise the medication and make sure he or she does not take an overdose.

HURTING ONESELF OR SWALLOWING THINGS

Self-injurious behavior occasionally occurs in foster children and disturbed children. It may be as simple as slamming a fist against the wall, or it may involve inflicting marks upon oneself or piercing body parts. The term "self-mutilation" is stronger than self-injury and implies that there is permanent damage. Ear piercing is not considered self-injurious.

These children may slash themselves or mark themselves persistently, and the results are infected wounds and large scars. Children who mutilate themselves are more often girls than boys. Studies indicate that about half of these children have been abused in the past. Children who injure themselves sometimes describe this as a need to ease their inner pain by hurting themselves on the outside.

Other forms of self-injury involve swallowing nonfood items. When children do this on purpose, they may swallow batteries, coins, or buttons. Although these may not be suicidal gestures, they indicate a wish to hurt oneself. Whatever the reason for self-injurious behavior, the result is immediate attention. This behavior cannot be ignored. If you have a foster child who punctures his or her own skin, clean the area. Consider the need for stitches and for a tetanus shot. Any child who swallows a foreign object needs to be evaluated in an emergency room.

There is no simple treatment for self-injurious behavior and no medication will prevent it. Self-injurious behavior is sometimes a part of depression and may represent a "cry for help" in a child who is considering suicide. This condition should always be discussed with the child's caseworker and other professionals.

RUDENESS IN FOSTER CHILDREN

It is a common complaint that many foster children just "don't seem very nice." Rudeness may develop in these children for logical reasons. Good manners are taught to most children by loving parents, who expect the child to learn to speak in a friendly manner from an early age. Foster children may have missed that part of development. Their biological familes may not have expected friendliness, or the family may not have paid much attention to this aspect of child rearing.

Also friendliness may not have worked for this child. This child may have asked politely for breakfast and not gotten it. As a foster child, he may ask politely to go back to his biological parents and the request is not granted. So he may feel that people pay little attention to a child who is quiet and well behaved. Also, children who are discouraged with life and uneasy about the future may express their worries by becoming unpleasant. They may not be sophisticated enough to tell you that they are worried.

So there are often good reasons for rudeness and bad manners in these children. However, the child will be more successful if he develops more pleasant behavior. In a younger child, foster parents should ignore bad manners and praise good manners. Indicate that shouting and yelling are not acceptable. A younger child will often learn quickly that rudeness is not appropriate in your home.

For an older child, these habits may not go away easily. Talk to the child about the way he interacts with others and suggest some changes in his behavior. Then, if that brings good results, point out the benefit of good manners. Work together with the teacher to find ways to discourage rudeness and encourage good manners.

Criticizing a child seldom cures rudeness. Providing a loving and consistent atmosphere is the best approach. When pleasant words from a foster child result in pleasant responses, he will feel less need to have loud and unpleasant ways.

MILD TO MODERATE DISRUPTIVE BEHAVIOR

Professionals call mild to moderate disruptive behavior "oppositional" or defiant behavior. As a foster parent, you might think of this as being argumentative, yelling, and not following rules. This behavior is a little more serious than rudeness.

An oppositional child may defy adults over rules. This child may appear to be still in the "terrible twos," although he or she is much older. These children often take a strong stand on issues, such as wanting to go to the mall, and then are unable to back down. If they lose an argument, they may sulk, complain, and disturb those around them.

Foster families can be quite helpful with oppositional children by providing opportunities for healthy social interaction. If possible, play board games and participate with the child in outdoor activities. Offer an occasional treat, such as a late night television program, for good behavior. Encourage the child to relax and laugh about things. Find something about the child that is attractive to you and to others. Maybe she is good at music, at styling hair, or at cooking. Encourage activities that allow her to interact with others in a positive way.

Many of these children benefit by physical activity and by the discipline of a sport. They may not be good at team sports, but track, martial arts, or some other sport that one does alone may work well for them. Bicycle riding with a foster parent is an example of a physical activity that may really help such a child.

"Every time they moved me, I made it my job to cause trouble," said one former foster child. "It got to be like a game. With each move, I'd stay in a foster home a shorter time. Then I got to a foster home where the family said I didn't need to go. They said they liked me a lot, even though my behavior was terrible. You know I continued to act bad for almost two years? Somehow, my foster parents put up with it. Now I'm in junior college."

Foster parents, biological parents, caseworkers, judges, and school personnel are all disturbed by an oppositional child. Unfortunately, studies show that most of these children do not do well and many go on to a life of juvenile delinquency or crime. Oppositional behavior may turn into more serious types of misbehavior, and such a child may get into trouble with the law.

Oppositional children are challenging for foster parents. Some foster parents are specifically trained for handling this type of behavior. The caseworker and the biological family should be involved in the care of such a child. The child who is oppositional is lucky if she finds a home where foster parents love her. Yet, this does happen, and oppositional behavior can begin to turn around in connection with a loving adult.

MODERATE TO SEVERE DISRUPTIVE BEHAVIOR

Child psychiatrists use the term "conduct disorder" for children whose behavior is so troubled that it affects others around them. The diagnosis is only used if the problem has gone on for many months. Children with conduct disorder commit acts that are harmful to others, such as stealing, fire-setting, and robbery. They may demonstrate cruelty to animals or to other people. They are unable to function in a useful way in society.

This type of behavior often results from the lifestyle the child has grown up in. Discipline has been weak and the child has not had rules to follow. He has received so little love and attention that he has no ability to care about others. In fact, it is all right with him to make others uncomfortable or to cause pain.

Foster parents should consider the child's background and the culture in which he was raised. Shoplifting and fighting may have been a way of life. However, the child needs to change this lifestyle if he wants to stay out of detention or jail. If you see signs of deep-seated trouble in his activities, talk to the child and the caseworker about future consequences if this behavior continues.

As you get to know this child, continue to explore his strengths and good qualities. Encourage the child to change and point out how his good moments lead to success. If a child is beginning to get into trouble, has set fires, is not going to school, or has hurt someone, the chances are that he will end up becoming a juvenile delinquent unless you and the caseworker can bring about change.

Find a psychologist or psychiatrist who can work with this child. That may require some looking. If the child has underlying hyperactivity or depression, he may need medication. He may need an evaluation for possible seizure disorder. Psychiatrists often try different medications to help such a child gain control over his life.

MEDICATIONS FOR ABNORMAL BEHAVIOR

Several different types of abnormal behavior have been examined in this chapter. Medication may be used for these children, and it may be prescribed by a pediatrician, a family practice doctor, or a psychiatrist.

The medications used for hyperactive behavior are actually adult stimulants. In such a child, the medication tends to lengthen the attention span and slow down the fidgeting. Medications for anxiety and nervousness are very commonly used in adults but are used sparingly in children. Antihistamines are often used to calm a child. Antipsychotic drugs, which are used for mentally disturbed adults, are sometimes used for abnormal behavior in children. They may help a child control himself during the day and help with sleep at night. The newer antipsychotics seem to be quite safe.

All medications have side effects, and your doctor should explain specific side effects of the medications prescribed. The pharmacist can also be helpful. If you feel the medication is causing any problems, call the doctor to discuss your concerns. Many of the medications used for behavior cause constipation, dryness of the mouth, and weight gain. Have the child drink plenty of liquids and limit food intake if possible.

Medication is only effective if it is taken regularly. Children are usually not able to manage their own medications. Keep containers up high and locked when not being used. If supplies get low, be sure to get refills. Watch the child taking the medication; if you are especially concerned, ask him to "open up" after swallowing, so you can be sure it went down.

Make arrangements for medication at school, camp, and on home visits. If the child is expected to leave your care, make sure there is a supply of his medication and that it is clear where to go for more medication and when there are return appointments.

PROFESSIONAL HELP FOR CHILDREN WITH
ABNORMAL BEHAVIOR

The abnormal behaviors described in this chapter can have serious consequences for the child and for the foster family. Making some changes in such a child's behavior is difficult, but efforts to do so are worthwhile. Most libraries and bookstores have books about troubled children, and reading several books will give you a balanced view.

Most foster parents begin a search for professional help with the caseworker. Your agency may call such a person a counselor, rather than a caseworker. The caseworker, the teacher, and the physician are all available for advice and guidance. Talk to each before deciding where to turn next. The school may have a behavior specialist who can help you. That person can work together with the child's doctor regarding medication, tests, and referrals to medical specialists.

Your caseworker may or may not be a social worker. If he or she is not and wishes to help you find a social worker, that would be appropriate. A social worker will probably want to talk to the teacher, the biological family, the child, the caseworker, and the foster parents. Any plan devised to help a child with seriously abnormal behavior will need input from all of these persons.

A psychologist is usually an expert on behavior. Sometimes a psychologist will do an initial evaluation and another person will continue to work with the child. On the other hand, some psychologists are available for ongoing help and may arrange weekly visits with the child. Psychiatrists may be needed to make a psychiatric diagnosis, to prescribe psychiatric drugs, or to arrange for further help in the mental health field. It is unusual that a psychiatrist would be involved on a weekly basis to follow a child, but that might be arranged.

The important thing is to find someone in these helping professions who can relate to the child. This professional will also need to work comfortably with all other members of the team.

A SAFE HOME FOR A CHILD WITH ABNORMAL BEHAVIOR

The abnormal behaviors described in this chapter may make safety an issue. You may be concerned about the safety of the foster child, your own safety and that of your family, or dangerous situations that might develop at school or in the community.

Safety rules that are appropriate for any foster family are even more important for families caring for children with abnormal behavior. Certain things should be locked and kept up high. This includes all lighters, all matches, all cash, all car keys, all medications, all guns, and all alcohol. Have a limited number of keys for these locked areas and keep the keys in your pocket.

Install extra smoke alarms and change the batteries every year. Check smoke alarms twice a year when you change your clocks. Do not assume any hiding place is safe. Do not hide things under your bed or in your sock drawer. Store valuables in a bank deposit box.

If you are quite concerned about a child, do not allow him to be in your home alone. Make sure you know where he is all day. Have the school call and tell you if he is absent.

VERY YOUNG TROUBLED CHILDREN

If you feel that a very young foster child is headed for some of the abnormal behavior described in this chapter, do not overdo the discipline. A young foster child, below the age of eight, who is oppositional may just be testing you and testing himself. Try to react in quiet ways without showing extreme displeasure, and praise the child when you approve of his actions. Most foster parents consider troubled children up to the age of about ten as able to make changes.

Safety rules are quite important with young children. They are more likely to play with a match or a gun than to mean harm in their actions. Still, these items must not be available to them. Young children whose behavior seems abnormal should never be left alone. If that is difficult for you, ask the caseworker to arrange respite care for the child. Such a child may need to be in another level of foster care, where there are specially trained foster parents. Institutional care may also be necessary for a short time.

RAISING A CHILD WITH ABNORMAL BEHAVIOR

For the majority of foster children, you should raise the child just as you did your own. The foster child will respond to your love and attention by becoming civilized and pleasant. However, children described in this chapter need special approaches from foster parents. The abnormal behavior is of several general types. Depression is one type, hyperactivity is a second, and disruptive behavior is a third. In each case, if a child is not raised with careful attention to problems, she may end up in serious trouble.

Most experts agree that a child who has one of the disruptive behavior problems, such as oppositional behavior or conduct disorder, needs to be handled with a fairly rigid structure. In some communities such children are sent to military schools or boot camps where discipline is quite tough. Your rules must be very clear to the child and you must pay close attention to whether or not rules are being followed. On a regular basis, you need to point out the consequences of misbehavior. If you feel that this child will soon be in trouble with the police, tell her that.

When pleasant times are arranged for such a child, you need to be constantly watching that this child is behaving in an acceptable manner. She is not able to monitor her own behavior well and if you do not watch her, there may be trouble. Read to her from the newspaper about young people who have succeeded and young people who have ruined their lives by being violent or cruel to others. Talk about good sportsmanship and good manners.

Sometimes these children, as they become older teenagers, simply drift out of foster care. They either return to their biological families or begin to live with friends or on the street. A child then becomes susceptible to the criminal lifestyle, may develop illnesses, and will not be able to be employed.

TEENS AND ABNORMAL SEXUALITY

The children described as oppositional or with conduct disorders have trouble relating to others. Boys with these problems see little reason not to seduce young women to have sex with them. They may try to sexually attract foster family members, schoolmates, or other young persons in their lives. They may force themselves on someone, resulting in serious problems with the police.

Boys who are sexually active and who are also undisciplined and have poor judgment may get their female partners pregnant. They are also likely to get and to pass on sexually transmitted diseases. HIV/AIDS is an obvious concern for such a child and his sexual partners.

Many schools and agencies have programs to help youngsters, both boys and girls, understand their own sexuality. These might consist of weekly sessions, for several weeks, and would cover ways to prevent pregnancy and disease transmission. For boys who have already tried to force their sexual attentions on others, called "sexual perpetrators," special groups are available.

Girls with these abnormal behaviors often see no reason not to have sex with multiple partners. The inhibitions that most young women have might be missing for these girls. They may give little thought to possible pregnancy or infection. In fact, pregnancy may sound attractive to them. Classes and programs on sexuality may be quite helpful for these young women. As you counsel them on the consequences of unprotected sex, you should probably concentrate on the risk of infection rather than the risk of pregnancy.

THE FUTURE FOR CHILDREN WITH ABNORMAL BEHAVIOR

The behaviors that have been described in this chapter are very disturbing for a foster family. Yet, there are many such children who need to find substitute parents to love them and take care of them. These children may have been in psychiatric institutions or involved in the juvenile justice system. They may have either of these placements ahead of them. Foster parents must make sure that they are comfortable with accepting such a child.

Most foster parents deal with a child with abnormal behavior by essentially having a contract with the agency and the child, indicating that they will keep the child as long as behavior is acceptable. This approach will work well if the child becomes fond of you, because it will maintain the focus on keeping better behavior. You may be prepared to forgive a few indiscretions; however, do not let the child know that.

What are the outcomes for these children? What will happen to them in the end? Some professionals feel that most of the problems described in this chapter are chronic and untreatable. A child who has been stealing, who has been skipping school, or who has been in detention may be on a slippery slide towards a life of crime. Some foster parents, however, feel that they can recognize an occasional resilient child from among these troubled adolescents. They feel that the love, encouragement, and consistent discipline they provide will change a child for the better.

12

Juvenile Delinquency and Juvenile Justice

This chapter is about foster children who get into trouble with the law. Unfortunately, it is not unusual for this to happen. The family difficulties that lead to foster placement of children may also lead to juvenile delinquency.

Research on criminal behavior has attempted to find the reasons for this behavior. Poverty is a factor. Drugs and alcohol are important, as a person who is impaired has probably lost judgment about right and wrong. Impulsiveness and depression are both mental problems that seem to lead to criminal activity. All of these factors are often referred to as stresses, and a combination of stresses seems to lead to illegal behavior.

Research on adult criminals has shown that many of them were abused as children and many of them were in foster care as children. That information suggests the value of trying to prevent foster children from misbehaving. If a foster child gets into trouble, foster parents need to understand the various legal situations that may arise. The legal system for children in trouble, called "juvenile justice," varies from state to state. These laws are currently changing, and there is a trend towards stricter laws and stricter law enforcement for misbehaving children.

GETTING IN TROUBLE WITH THE LAW

Adolescents, whether or not they are foster children, may drink alcohol, stay out late at night, or skip school. As a foster parent, whenever this type of testing behavior occurs, you should say, "I love you and I do not like your behavior." The child needs to be told that the behavior is wrong and that it has consequences. You may create these consequences or the consequences may involve the police and the court system.

Usually, the first brush with the law occurs when an adolescent or teenager is brought into the police station for a minor offense. Police will call the parents when they bring a child to the station. If you get such a call, contact the caseworker and then go to the police station. The police can release a child without going to court. The child may get a lecture and may be warned that the next time there is trouble, he or she will have to go to court.

If a child continues to behave badly, he or she will probably have a petition filed to the juvenile justice system. The probation department may be asked to do a study of home and school and then will report to the court. At this stage, the child may still not have to go to court. Probation officers may set some ground rules, such as school attendance and staying drug-free. The child may be told that if he or she breaks these ground rules he or she will go to court.

On the other hand, a child may be sent to court to appear before the judge. If possible, go to court with the child. Usually family court judges or juvenile court judges take a parent-like position. Listen carefully to what the judge says so that you can reinforce it later.

You should always expect good behavior from a foster child. Never indicate to the child that bad behavior is expected because of his or her birth family. You should expect the child to be law-abiding. Also, never make excuses like "boys will be boys." You may hope that the child will outgrow this behavior, but never indicate that you are confident that the behavior will pass. Just like any parent, you need to continue to say that you love the child but cannot tolerate the behavior.

JUVENILE JUSTICE

Illegal acts committed by youngsters are called "offenses" rather than crimes. The juvenile justice system deals with children accused of committing offenses. Each state has different rules. The age a person is no longer a juvenile also varies. In many states, that occurs at age eighteen.

The judges in this system (juvenile court judges or family court judges) have more choices than in regular courts. There is no jury and no formal trial structure. Children are evaluated by the probation department before going to court. Trials in this system are called hearings. Before going to court, a child may be ordered to stay in detention. Detention facilities do not house adults, only youths. The average stay in detention before going to court is about two weeks.

Detention also may be used as a punishment. Other facilities where young people are incarcerated are called training schools, camps, or group homes. A child usually is incarcerated less than a year. These facilities are similar to adult correctional facilities, such as jail or prison. There is a no-nonsense approach to trying to improve a child's behavior. "We try to find a balance between love and discipline," said a staff member in a detention facility. "We try to prepare them for a life in the mainstream instead of a future behind bars."

A juvenile delinquent has committed an offense that would have been a criminal act for an adult. If the judge decides that a child did commit an offense, the child may be sent to detention for a period of time. If the child is not sentenced to serve time in detention, the youngster may need to follow certain rules, perform community service, or pay back the victim.

If a child is accused of a serious crime, like murder, that child may be moved into the adult criminal system. In that case, there is a formal trial and the child has the same rights as an adult who is tried for a crime.

CHILDREN'S OFFENSES (STATUS OFFENSES)

"Status offenses" are specific to children and include ungovernability, truancy, running away, and being out at night. These offenses would not be considered crimes if committed by an adult. Although status offenses may seem minor, such an offense may be the beginning of future criminal involvement for a child.

If a nonfoster child is found guilty of a status offense, he or she may be determined to be in need of supervision by the court. Such a designation may be called PINS or CHINS. Sometimes, if a child is placed under court supervision, he or she will be removed from home. Such a youngster may enter a foster home at that time, under court supervision.

In all likelihood, such a foster child would like to go back home. The judge may set certain requirements for the child, such as good school attendance and staying drug-free. If the child meets the requirements, the judge will consider allowing the child to return home. Some foster parents have a special interest in this type of child.

A child like this, an offender who has not committed a serious crime, may have abnormal behavior and that behavior may make it likely that there will be further illegal acts. Such a child would benefit by guidance from a psychiatrist or psychologist. Medication may be quite effective.

A mental health clinic may offer a variety of services for youthful offenders who have behavior problems. Classes and evening sessions may allow children to get together with others who have similar problems. The youth may learn from one another and also be guided by professionals.

PROBATION AND THE PROBATION DEPARTMENT

The probation department is involved in most family court or juvenile court cases. The probation officer will visit the school and the home, interview the family and the child, and determine whether or not a petition needs to be filed to have the child brought to court.

If a petition is filed, then adjudication and disposition are the events that will occur in court. In both cases the probation officer will be there.

"Adjudication" is the judge's decision on whether the youth is guilty. "Disposition" is the judge's decision on punishment. The probation department will make sure that the judge's requirements are understood and that they are followed.

The judge may sentence the child to a period of probation. During probation, the person has conditional freedom and must meet certain requirements in order to stay out of a correctional or detention facility. If the child was in foster care before going to court, he or she will probably remain in foster care as part of the disposition.

The probation department is supposed to keep in close contact with children who have been in trouble and make sure that their behavior is improving. A probation officer may have significant influence on decisions that are made by the judge. Problems occur because, in general, probation officers do not have time to monitor each child closely.

TRUANCY OR SKIPPING SCHOOL

Truancy is being late to school or not attending school. It is only of concern in children, since adults are not required to attend school. Truancy is not a crime, but it is an offense that will cause a child to be brought before the authorities. If a child is truant without an excuse for a period of time, the school will report the child to the probation department. Someone, perhaps a probation officer, will talk to the child and family. The child may be required to improve his or her attendance in order to avoid going to court.

Skipping school may start in young children. If a young foster child wants to skip school and asks your permission, the answer should be no. Many foster parents have a rule about school attendance, such as "children always go to school unless they are sick." In adolescents, skipping school is often an early sign of trouble. In most states, persistent truancy is a status offense under the age of sixteen. Truancy leads to dropping out of high school. Experts in law enforcement call truancy a "gateway crime," because children who are not occupied in school tend to get into trouble.

If a child is an older teenager and has been skipping school, he or she may be unhappy in school. Try to find out what is going on. Consider the need for a different educational program. Talk to school personnel and see if they have special methods to encourage attendance. The foster child who goes to court for truancy risks a change in placement. He or she might be sent to another foster home or to an institution.

VERY YOUNG CHILDREN WHO GET INTO TROUBLE

When children under the age of ten get into trouble, they usually come from extremely difficult home situations. About half of these children have a parent in jail. Most of these children have been neglected or abused.

Firesetting may be the most common "crime" committed by children under ten. Usually the child did not set out to do harm to anyone. However, the safeguards that are normally in place to keep very young children safe were not there. Often the very young child who commits an offense has no father, and the mother has left the child alone or has gone to sleep while the child is awake. That child may leave home and commit offenses with little motivation.

Although there is a movement in the United States to consider the very young offender a criminal, these children usually remain protected from the adult justice system. They are usually not locked up. The judge often orders additional supervision of the child within the biological home or placement in foster care.

If you have a foster child under the age of ten who is getting into trouble with the police, try to find activities that will keep him occupied. Do not allow the child to be home alone or to be unsupervised within the home. After-school programs may be directed towards such children. Do not get too discouraged if such a child does continue to cause trouble. This is a difficult problem to solve. In general, the younger the offender, the more likely he will become a criminal as an adult.

FIRESETTING

Children often find fire exciting and fascinating. If interest in fire is kept within normal bounds, a child will grow up safely. For the occasional child, development is disturbed and abnormal interest in fire becomes a problem. Children who start fires are called "firesetters," not arsonists. In general, their interest is in gaining attention and causing excitement, rather than a malicious interest in seeing structures destroyed. Young firesetters come out of impoverished neighborhoods, from families with limited capabilities to parent them. There is no specific cure for this interest, which is so frightening to those around the child.

If a child comes into your home who has a history of firesetting, specific precautions should be taken. Check your smoke alarms. Install an extra smoke alarm in this child's bedroom. Remove the closet door, as that is where children usually set fires. Keep all lighters and matches up high and under lock and key. Make sure there are no secret collections of matches in another child's room.

Many fire departments have firemen especially trained to counsel such children. Look into that type of help. Never burn or scald a child in order to teach him a lesson. You must speak to the teacher about the child if there was firesetting in the past, as it is important for the safety of those in the school.

STEALING

Children who enter foster care often come from troubled families where stealing may have been a common activity. One way to help prevent stealing is to remember to praise a child for waiting, such as, "I knew you wanted a yo-yo and I'm so glad you waited until Friday." In addition, child care experts feel that the more loved and protected a child feels, the less likely he is to commit offenses such as stealing.

Even though you have tried to prevent it, the foster child may steal food, toys, or money. When questioned, such a child may say, "I never got anything myself so now I deserve to take it." This child is using his previous position as a victim as an excuse for victimizing others. Foster families should understand this reasoning but continue to point out to a foster child that it is not acceptable to steal.

Stealing among boys is quite common. It is estimated that 90 percent of boys steal at least once. However, whenever an episode of stealing occurs, the child must to be told that it is wrong, that there will be consequences, and that there needs to be repayment.

Stealing is usually the offense that takes a youngster into the category of a juvenile delinquent. Stealing, which may start out as a habitual behavior for a young foster child, may turn into true criminal behavior in a teenager. Stealing becomes a serious criminal act if there is a weapon.

AGGRESSION AND VIOLENT TENDENCIES

Many children, especially boys, get into fights with other children when they are four- to eight-years old. This behavior has a tendency to disappear, so that older boys seldom fight. If you have a foster child older than ten who gets into fights frequently, there is a potential for him to become more aggressive. With such a child, you must firmly put into place a "no fighting in my house" rule and enforce it. Do not let wrestling and jostling get started, because it may get out of hand.

When an aggressive gesture occurs, react to it. If you are too busy, tell the child you want to talk about it later. Sit down and try to figure out what made him angry. Try to talk the child through it, describing the consequences of the fight that might have developed. Then suggest some other ways he could have handled his feelings. Try to find a suggestion that satisfies the child.

Studies show several factors that seem to lead to violent behavior. First, television and movies have presented violent behavior as "normal" for this generation of children. You need to tell children that movies do not represent reality. Point out violence that would have caused heartache and a jail sentence in real life. Talk about going to court and going to jail.

Second, there are weapons in many households. A foster child should never have access to weapons. Ideally, a foster home should have no weapons, and if there are guns, they should be kept up high, locked, and unloaded. A third factor is that foster children may have been raised in violent households. Guns and other weapons may have been part of family life.

There may have been real-life occurrences where someone tried to settle a problem by hitting or shooting.

There are currently specific concerns about violence in schools. If a child is angry at a teacher, you and the child should visit the principal. It would be helpful to try to resolve situations where a child has a great deal of anger towards a teacher or another student.

Violent activity is often not a solitary act. There is often a group of boys who encourage and dare each other to perform illegal actions. This group may or may not be a true gang, but the peer pressure of a child's friends urging him may be quite effective for a foster child.

If a foster child is aggressive or violent, if he hurts others, he will be sent to juvenile court or family court. Very likely, if the problem has gone on for several months, he will be removed from your home and put into detention or a residential treatment center. Make sure that the child knows these consequences.

JUVENILE DELINQUENCY

If a child has committed a serious offense, a family court judge or juvenile court judge may say that a child is a juvenile delinquent. A child is not designated a juvenile delinquent if he has committed a noncriminal offense such as trespassing. Neither will he be termed a juvenile delinquent for commission of a status offense, such as truancy.

Juvenile delinquents have been found guilty of a misdemeanor or a felony. In most cases, the family court judge or juvenile court judge will handle this type of crime without a jury. The young person may be sentenced to detention for a period of time, or he may be sent back home on probation. The child who is a juvenile delinquent will be watched over by a judge until he has grown up.

In rare cases, a child suspected of having committed a severe felony will be tried as an adult. Then the child will enter the adult criminal system. Trial will occur, as for an adult, and the youth may be sentenced to an adult prison.

If your foster child is accused or suspected of a misdemeanor or felony, there will be many issues ahead. You need to be in close contact with caseworker and birth parents. Can the child stay with you until a trial? Will the child be able to return to you after serving time in detention? These are difficult questions.

If you love this foster child and if you have been a good foster parent, then you should stay involved, just like any family member. Try to visit the child and go to court when the child goes to court.

FOSTER PROGRAMS FOR CHILDREN WHO ARE IN TROUBLE

There are some foster homes that specialize in taking in youths from the juvenile justice system. These families provide specialized care with special

training. Children usually come and go every few weeks. Since they are allowed to stay in this level of care only if they behave well, this provides an
incentive to stay out of trouble. Foster families who take offenders into their
homes generally have rather strict rules and schedules. Law enforcement
officers or probation officers usually monitor these children carefully.

Research suggests that such children might benefit by a period in a specialized foster home. The youth is removed from the birth family and the
neighborhood, which may be beneficial. Structured programs that try to
change the youngster's attitude and behavior seem to work and to decrease offending behavior. There is no evidence that periods of incarceration have a positive effect on a child's behavior. Old-fashioned psychiatric
care, which involved discussing the reasons for misbehavior, is also not
effective.

Many times these youths in trouble with the law turn out to be pleasant
children who just need a lot of attention and help. You may be a person who
can provide the structure and the love that these children need. The rewards of helping such a child can be great.

ILLEGAL DRUGS AND PROSTITUTION

As foster children grow into the late teenage years, they often realize that
their financial situation is dismal. They have no money and no family structure to help them get a start in life. So they will seek ways to make money,
and they may take significant risks in illegal activities.

When foster children get into trouble, very often drugs are involved.
That does not usually mean that the youngster is addicted. Rather, a foster
child who is involved with drugs is usually selling them to make money.
Young people are often used in the drug trade and, although the risks are
great, the money comes easily.

Prostitution means getting paid to have sex. That is also very common,
once a child is involved with people who use and sell drugs. It is, unfortunately, a way young people feel that they can make money. Again, the risks
are significant.

Selling drugs and being a prostitute both have health and safety risks.
For either activity, the danger of HIV/AIDS and the possibility of gunshot
injuries are very real. Both activities are also illegal, and a child who is
caught may end up going to detention or jail.

TEENS WHO COMMIT MURDER AND GO ON
SHOOTING SPREES

Some murders occur as part of a violent lifestyle. A young person who
steals or who is involved in drugs may murder someone without giving it a
lot of thought. Such crimes are unpremeditated, meaning that the child did

not put a complicated plan in place. Victims of these murders may be family, friends, or neighborhood enemies. Murderer and victim may have a quite similar lifestyle.

When a young person is a murder suspect, the case will usually be moved into the adult criminal system. This system allows the child to have a legal defense and a jury. The child will be found either guilty or innocent. If innocent, he may go free. If guilty, the young person will go to jail or prison.

Another type of murder committed by teenagers that seems to be a fairly recent development is a "shooting spree." With little or no warning, these youngsters have gone into schools or other public areas and started shooting. Similar events have resulted from the use of explosives. The only understanding of reasons for these attacks is that the murderer was "angry." Long periods of planning may occur before the attack actually happens.

These occurrences result in tremendous publicity. Other youngsters see the excitement and understand that the murder was committed because of anger. Such children recognize that anger, feel that such an attack might bring them satisfaction, and then additional shootings occur.

Anger has always been part of the teenage lifestyle. Gangs form for protection against the anger of other gangs. Teenage anger is also expressed toward parents and other authorities. In these cases, the teen often seems to feel that parents have not allowed him to be independent enough.

There is no indication that foster children are any more likely to go on "shooting sprees" than other children. In fact, most foster children do not have the ability to make the kind of complicated plans that generally precede these events. These crimes do not seem to be caused by poverty. Little is known about prevention of this type of violence. The secretive nature of the preparation makes it difficult for parents to know what is going on.

13

Common Health-Related Problems in Foster Children

There are certain health-related problems common in children from troubled homes. In some cases, poor parenting skills or lack of attention may have caused a child to have a problem that should have been outgrown. In other situations, the child's health has been neglected. Problems such as dental cavities and poor vision can be identified and corrected while the child is in foster care.

All of the problems discussed below are common in troubled homes where poverty and other stresses are factors. Placement in a loving foster home may help, and some of these problems will disappear naturally. However, in other cases, foster parents should seek treatment. All of these concerns are everyday issues for pediatricians. Be sure to consult with the child's doctor or other professionals at the child's clinic.

DELAYS IN TALKING

Speech delay is common if children grow up in homes where there is confusion, poverty, and neglect. If parents have not been talking to the child, speech will not develop normally. All children, especially foster children, benefit from lots of talking and listening in the home. Reading to a child is important and having an older child read aloud is a good way to encourage language development in that child. Singing is a useful way to help children learn to talk. It is fine to repeat yourself when talking with children. Saying things over and over may be comforting to a child who is quite young.

If the child continues to have slow speech, talk to the child's doctor and to the caseworker. You may be advised to talk to officials at the school and ask for an evaluation. If speech therapy is needed, there will be a special meeting to make arrangements. Be sure to go to the meeting. One foster mother said, "I always take Tasha to the meetings. I think it helps the school officials to know that she's a real kid and she's got real problems. I usually get what she needs, that way."

Your foster child may have been in a speech program elsewhere. The caseworker can help arrange for continuation or for a different program if necessary. A preschooler can get speech therapy either in a preschool setting or in the home. If speech therapy is recommended, try to be present at some of the sessions. The therapist will suggest special activities to do at home. A child's language will improve faster if everyone works together with the same approaches.

Older children may not want to go to speech therapy. Often the therapist and child decide to stop speech therapy by the time a child is ten or eleven years old. Even without formal speech therapy, foster families can be quite effective in encouraging a child to learn new words and new ways of talking. At the same time, it is important to be accepting of a child who has a different way of talking. With older children, continue to use reading aloud as an excellent way of encouraging language development.

HEARING PROBLEMS

Deafness, in its more severe forms, is a serious disability. It may not be recognized in babies, especially if family life is confusing. When a new foster baby comes into your home, take a few quiet moments to assure yourself that her hearing is adequate. Whisper in the baby's ear to see if she turns toward the sound.

If there is a question about your foster baby's hearing, speak to the child's doctor. Testing can be arranged, although there is no easy test that will prove that a child can hear. Talk to the doctor about whether the child is "tuning you out." Conditions such as autism or mental retardation may cause a child to be unable to communicate even though hearing is adequate.

If a baby has had a prolonged stay in the newborn nursery, prematurity or other problems may have affected hearing. Also, if there were frequent ear infections in the past, hearing may have been impaired. Child abuse and head injury may cause hearing loss.

An older child should have a hearing test done regularly at school. If you have concerns, call the school nurse to inquire about testing. Even with an older child, behavior may get in the way of responding to an adult's voice. Hearing clinics can evaluate such a child. Sometimes they report slowness of processing, indicating that you should allow more time for your words to get through to the child.

A deaf or hearing-impaired child will qualify for special services. Hearing aides may be used. The child may need to sit at the front of the classroom. Sign language or other special methods of communication may be taught. A special classroom or a special school may be necessary.

DELAYS IN PHYSICAL DEVELOPMENT

Normally a child should walk on his own by fifteen months of age. A few more months can be allowed for a foster child. However, if a child is eighteen-months old and is not walking, you should talk to the child's doctor. Other development may also be delayed, such as learning to dress and feed himself.

As a foster parent, consider whether a child who has motor delays seems to be mentally normal. If that is the case, the doctor will consider cerebral palsy or muscular dystrophy as possible causes of the physical problem. If mental development also seems slow, and language is slow, the child may be mentally retarded.

Children who have been neglected or abused will probably not develop normally. Often there is a mixture in such a child of early independence and also of delays. Psychologists who evaluate young children who have been abused often note this type of mixed development. Such children have the potential to overcome their delays as they begin to live in a more natural environment.

Whatever the case, physical delay in children should always lead to an evaluation by appropriate professionals. Physical and occupational therapy may help such children improve their motor skills.

ABNORMAL EATING HABITS

Foster children may be picky eaters. Teaching a child to try new foods takes time and patience. If you are worried that the child is not eating enough, ask the doctor if her weight is normal and how much she should be gaining. Then have the child weighed again in a few months. Children who enter foster care are often small and there may be catch-up growth in the first year or two.

Some foster children have gone hungry in the past. You may notice them gorging themselves and they may hide food in their bedrooms. Their table manners may be poor. Such a child will probably develop better eating habits after a few weeks in foster care. However, the child's memory of hunger may continue to be disturbing.

Some foster children eat large amounts and gain excessive weight. Check with the doctor before getting too concerned. Weight gain may be normal for a healthy adolescent. If a child becomes overweight in your care, do not consider it a failure on your part. Obesity is a problem for many Americans and it usually starts during childhood or adolescence. Medication used for behavior problems may cause excessive weight gain.

If a child literally refuses to eat and seems to be on a hunger strike, keep a close eye on her, but do not insist that she eat. The child may eat a little when you are not confronting her. Make sure she drinks liquids. Call the doctor and caseworker when the child cannot hear you and discuss the problem. Let the doctor decide when to take action.

Anorexia nervosa and bulimia are unusual in foster children. These eating disorders tend to occur in adolescent girls who want to be thin. Youngsters with anorexia refuse to eat and they lose weight. Bulimia causes purposeful vomiting after eating. These behaviors need the help of professionals for diagnosis and treatment.

"Pica" is a term for eating nonfood items. Children may chew on paper or other harmless material. If a child eats chips of paint or plaster, the child's blood lead level may become elevated. Lead poisoning affects intelligence, so if you are concerned, ask the doctor to do a blood test for lead. Watch young children closely if they put small objects in their mouths. They may swallow or inhale the objects and the result may be quite serious.

DIETARY CONCERNS FOR FOSTER CHILDREN

It may be challenging to change a foster child's eating habits. She has had a lifetime of learning to eat certain foods, prepared in certain ways. Unless the child is a teenager, she will be eating mainly in your home. Do not buy junk food. Buy fruit and other healthful snacks. Do not buy carbonated beverages for routine use.

If a child comes from a different cultural background from yours, inquire into the child's previous eating habits. Try to include some of her favorite items in your meal plans. You may need to adapt recipes so that the food is healthful. Often it is the spices that actually make for the differences in ethnic food style.

A healthy diet for American children is to get plenty of starch, vegetables, and fruits. Starch includes potatoes, rice, bread, and pasta. There should be five servings of vegetables and fruits per day. Low-fat dairy products provide calcium, and protein needs are met with small servings of meat. Low-fat milk and low-fat yogurt should be standard in your house. It is important to not only provide a good diet, but to teach the foster child good judgment. Teach the child to buy healthy foods and prepare healthy meals.

A daily multivitamin supplement with iron is probably a good idea for foster children. If your water supply does not have fluoride added, get vitamin tablets that also contain fluoride. Talk to the doctor as a prescription may be necessary. Teenaged girls should definitely take a multivitamin with iron. The iron is appropriate for the blood loss of menstruation, and the vitamin supplement helps start good habits should she ever want to get pregnant.

If your foster child is overweight, it is certainly worth trying to help him or her to lose weight. Talk to the doctor or clinic and see if they can help you and the child set up a dietary program. Remember that overweight children may only need to maintain their weight because they will grow taller. Such a child needs to increase his or her exercise. Studies indicate that excessive television watching is associated with excessive weight gain in children.

BEDWETTING

Wetting the bed is very common in young children, especially boys. It is normal to wet the bed at night, up to the age of five. Most foster parents are not surprised by bedwetting. They put plastic sheets on the bed and tell the child not to worry. It is important not to shame or punish the child.

If bedwetting occurs in a child who has been dry in the past, consider a urinary tract infection. Talk to the doctor and see if a urine specimen is indicated. In addition, constipation can cause urinary accidents.

Make sure the child can get quickly to the bathroom and that he can unfasten his pajamas. Also, make sure he is not afraid to get up alone. Turn on a night-light. Talk about how nice it would be if he got up and went to the bathroom at night. If the child is willing to restrict fluid intake, have him stop drinking liquids a few hours before bedtime. Try getting him up once before you go to bed. You may be able to walk or carry him, even if half asleep, to the bathroom to urinate. Once the child has had a dry bed for a while, he may begin to get up at night by himself.

Most children eventually outgrow this problem. If it persists, talk to the doctor. There are medications that can be used, but they do not offer lasting benefit. Talk to the child in a positive way. Tell the child that he or she will outgrow the problem, which will probably happen.

CONSTIPATION

Most children have a bowel movement every day or every two days. Children often cannot tell you if they have had a bowel movement because it does not seem important to them. If a child becomes cranky or unhappy and complains of a stomachache, he or she may be constipated. Constipation in children is common, particularly in boys, around the age of two or three. If toilet training has not gone smoothly, the child may resist sitting on the toilet and "hold in" the stool. Gradually, the fecal material becomes large and is difficult to evacuate. With this conditioning, called "encopresis," there may actually be soiling or diarrhea, as stool leaks around the mass.

If the child is constipated, you can give a nonprescription laxative in a child-sized dose. Watch to see if he successfully has a bowel movement by the next day. Do not give enemas or suppositories unless the doctor has recommended this, as children are frightened by these procedures. If constipation persists, call the doctor or clinic. There are some rare physical causes of constipation.

Once the problem has been resolved, keep the child on a high-fiber diet, which includes fruits and bran cereals. Make sure he drinks plenty of fluids. This will keep the bowels soft and help to prevent constipation. Also, set a time to go to the bathroom when no one else will bother the child. Praise him if he goes during that time. If he does not go, try again later in the day.

SLEEP PROBLEMS

Young children sleep more than older children. Babies often seem to need to cry a little before they go to sleep. They should not be put to sleep with a bottle. A young baby should always be put to sleep on her back or side. SIDS, or Sudden Infant Death Syndrome, seems to occur more often when babies sleep on their stomachs.

When a child is between eighteen and twenty-four months, she may begin to climb out of the crib. At that point, it is important to put the child into a low bed. Children can hurt themselves climbing out of a crib when the sides are up, and once they have learned to get out, they will continue to do so.

If an older foster child comes to your home, he or she may not have developed good sleeping habits. Be comforting if the child seems frightened. Sit with her, sing to her, and get her a small drink of milk or water. It may be important to have a favorite toy or blanket. Leave a door open or a light on. Going to sleep often frightens children, and this is especially true with foster children. Abuse or violence, if it occurred in the biological home, probably occurred in the night. Memories of these experiences can be disturbing even in the safety of a foster home. If the child wants to get into your bed, this is not necessarily bad. However, try not to let it become a habit.

Sleepwalking occurs in some young school-aged children. The child may silently walk around the house or even go outside. If there are night terrors the child will cry out, and the crying may be quite persistent. Try to make sure the child cannot get hurt. Usually these problems go away naturally.

VISION PROBLEMS

A child may come to you with glasses. Children generally are given glasses if they are near-sighted—that is, if they cannot see things well at a distance. When you go to the clinic for the child's first check-up, ask the doctor to measure the child's vision on an E-chart, with and without glasses. If there is a vision problem, take the child to an eye doctor. If glasses are recommended, be sure and ask when they need to be worn.

Sometimes a child arrives at a new foster home and says, "I'm supposed to have glasses, but I left them at the last place." The actual fact is that foster children often break or lose their glasses. Getting new glasses is seldom an emergency. Take time to get to know a child before going to the eye doctor. Then, when new glasses arrive, try keeping them in a drawer for part of the day.

If a young child appears to be cross-eyed and his eyes tend to turn in or out, be sure to make an appointment to have that checked. Poor vision in one eye may become permanent if the problem is not taken care of.

If a foster child has vision problems that cannot be corrected with glasses, the child will qualify for special services. Visually impaired or blind children need special schooling and special mobility training to move about. Equipment and technology is available to help the child read. Many communities have agencies that help take care of visually impaired persons.

DENTAL PROBLEMS

The most common dental problem that results from neglect is numerous dental cavities. If cavities are significant, you can usually see them when you look in the mouth. A large cavity may cause some cold or heat sensitivity or may become infected. However, sometimes children have large cavities and experience no discomfort.

If the child does not already have a dentist, try to take him to your own dentist. See if the dentist will accept the payment provided by the agency for a first visit, just to see what the child's dental needs are. Then, if there is expensive dental work that needs to be done, you may have to search for a dentist. Ask your family dentist or the child's doctor for a dental clinic that will accept payment for this child.

Do not cause undue fear of the dentist with these children. If you, yourself, are afraid of going to the dentist, do not share your anxiety with the child. If a child needs extensive dental work, try to help the child get through the experience without general anesthesia. It is always safer to keep a child awake, and most dental work done on children is not very painful.

The dentist or hygienist can be helpful in teaching good dental habits. Ask the dentist whether the child needs fluoride or any special brushing techniques. You can help young children have healthy teeth by avoiding candy and gum.

You may have an older foster child who has crooked teeth and needs braces. Remember that most children can skip braces during adolescence and have them in adulthood. However, young people with severely crooked teeth may need braces. You may be able to find a clinic where an orthodontist will accept whatever payment is available. Perhaps you can find a biological family member to pay for the braces. Call a local orthodontist's office and ask what special services might be available for a foster child.

SKIN PROBLEMS

A few minor skin problems are fairly common in children who have been neglected in the past. These problems usually clear up easily with good hygiene and some simple treatments.

Diaper rash may result from leaving diapers on too long. If a new baby comes to you with a rash, change the diaper frequently. Wash the area gently after a bowel movement. Keep the diaper off part of the time. Apply petroleum jelly for protection several times a day.

Dry skin may be worse in the winter. The skin all over the body will be scaly and may itch. Roughness of the hands and elbows is common. Dry skin can be treated with lotion, cold cream, or petroleum jelly applied all over the body, once a day. Eczema is an allergic skin rash that starts out with dry skin after which certain areas become inflamed. Common areas are around the ears, the elbows, and the knees. The skin may look thick and be darkly pigmented. Eczema may be itchy. It is treated with cold cream or petroleum jelly all over the body once a day. Also, use hydrocortisone cream once or twice a day on the itchy, inflamed areas. This condition is not contagious.

Acne is a facial condition of adolescents. It is more common in boys than girls. It causes red bumps on the face, and it can cause embarrassment. Treatment with nonprescription creams that contain benzoyl peroxide can be quite successful. The treatment is preventive, it does not make a pimple actually go away. Remind the child to use the treatment twice a day. Dietary factors are no longer considered important.

INACTIVE CHILD

It may seem odd that it is necessary to encourage children to exercise, but children are as likely as adults to be couch potatoes. Television is attractive to children and tends to keep them inside. Also, foster parents often want their foster children to stay close to home and not roam the neighborhood.

The benefits of exercise are only beginning to be understood. In adults, there is good evidence that regular exercise keeps blood pressure down, keeps weight down, and adds years of life expectancy. For children, an additional benefit is that physical activity during the day helps them to sit quietly and do homework in the evening. A child will be pointed in a good direction for a healthy and productive life if regular physical activity takes place every day.

Getting a foster child up and moving is best done by example. If someone in the family bikes or jogs, he or she should take the child along. If soccer is a family passion, get the child involved. If your family is not active, you will need to consider ways to get the foster child some exercise. At the same time, you may need to provide supervision, so that the child does not get into trouble. Besides the supervision issue, there may be a cost factor. So try to find an inexpensive activity that the child enjoys, one in which there is adult supervision, and make sure he or she gets there regularly.

DELAYED IMMUNIZATIONS

There are frequent changes in recommendations in this area, so for the most up-to-date information, talk to the doctor or clinic where your child goes. You can also talk to the school nurse, who can tell you what shots are required by the school. Some shots are merely recommended, but not required. However, most pediatricians would urge foster parents to get every available immunization for the foster child.

Traditional baby shots are for diphtheria, tetanus, pertussis, measles, mumps, rubella, and polio. These have been given for many years, so very likely your foster child has had them all. However, if there is no documentation, the shots may have to be repeated. This does not cause any harm, but it is an inconvenience. Also, boosters may be needed.

A fairly new immunization is the chickenpox (varicella) shot. While generally not required, it may be recommended for children who have not had the disease. Chickenpox is an unpleasant illness that has many complications, so it is good to give the vaccine to babies. If a foster child has come after early childhood, there may not be information about whether or not he had chickenpox. Talk to the biological mother, if appropriate, and then ask the doctor about the advisability of giving the chickenpox vaccine.

Hepatitis B is a devastating illness that tends to occur in poor communities. Hepatitis B vaccine is now used routinely in babies. It is administered in a series of three shots. If the child has gotten one or two, the series does not need to be restarted. However, there is no harm in getting extra doses of this vaccine. A diphtheria and tetanus booster is necessary every ten years and is usually due around the age of fifteen. A repeat measles-mumps-rubella shot might be given at the same time.

The requirements and recommendations for immunizations change from time to time and differ from state to state. The important thing is to get as much protection for the child as possible and then to keep good records. Keep a copy of your foster child's immunizations at your house.

A skin test for tuberculosis is often done in children from poor environments. If there is no swelling two days after the test, it is negative, and the child will probably not need another test for many years. If it is positive, talk to the doctor. A chest X ray and preventive treatment may be necessary.

MENSTRUAL PROBLEMS

A foster daughter may come to your home before starting to have menstrual periods. Menstruation usually begins around the age of twelve or about two years after the beginning of breast development. For the first year, periods may be irregular. Help the youngster learn to keep a record of her menstrual periods by marking a calendar.

Some young women have discomfort with their periods. Treatment recommended is to use ibuprofen every four to six hours. For persistent discomfort, birth control pills may be prescribed. The child does not need to change her level of activity during menstrual periods. Be sure she has the personal items she needs when she is away from home.

If a young girl is sexually active, it is possible for her to become pregnant even before starting to menstruate. After menstruation begins, pregnancy will be a concern for sexually active young women unless she uses protection. Education about sexual activity should begin in girls by the age of ten—earlier if breast development has already started. Make sure the child understands about sexual intercourse and the use of condoms. Offer to take her to a family planning clinic.

14

When the Child Is Ill
or Injured

All children get sick from time to time; however, a foster child may react to illness differently. Infections are the most common childhood illnesses. Injuries are also common and may occur frequently in foster children with poor safety habits and abnormal behavior.

Sometimes foster children have had a recurring medical problem, like frequent ear infections or urinary tract infections. Foster parents will need to gather information about such recurring problems. You should always be alert to possible allergies. The child may have had an allergy all along or a new allergy may arise. You need to help the child learn about this allergy.

It is important for foster children to know about their own illnesses and allergies. Foster children often need to carry their own medical information in their heads as they move from place to place.

MEDICAL RECORDS OF FOSTER CHILDREN

The agency you are working with will have given you some medical information on the foster child. You may be disappointed that it is not complete, but that is often unavoidable. Foster children may have records scattered in various clinics and various communities.

To start with, you need information about immunizations, allergies, and previous illnesses. If you cannot obtain that information from the agency or clinic, the school may be helpful. The biological family and previous foster parents also can help. Your agency may have a nurse who is responsible for records, and he or she can help in gathering together this type of information.

Be sure you keep good health records of all foster children. Make a copy of the immunization record and store it away in a permanent place. Whenever there is a visit to a clinic or dentist, make a note about it and put that note in the child's folder.

If the foster child is old enough to understand, he or she should be fully informed about any health care concerns. There is no guarantee that written information will stay with the child. If possible tell the child that he or she can call you after moving on if information is needed.

DEALING WITH A SICK FOSTER CHILD

Even if the foster child is old enough to stay home alone, do not allow her to stay home alone the first few times she is ill. You do not know the child well enough to know how she will react to illness. Plan to spend some time with the child. You may be the first adult who has ever cared for her, during an illness, and it may be a valuable lesson that people expect to take care of each other.

Make sure the child is comfortable. Do not be surprised if she exaggerates her symptoms. Keep a close eye on her, but try not to indicate that you are worried. Pay special attention to symptoms that you can verify, such as fever or swelling.

Your foster child may relish the time alone with you in a quiet house. This is appropriate, as the child probably has missed such quiet times with her own parents. Provide chicken soup and pamper the child for the first few illnesses, then expect her to get through later illnesses without as much special attention.

If the child is new to you and becomes sick enough to see a doctor, this may be a good experience for both of you. If possible, do not send the child to the doctor with a caseworker. You are the substitute parent and she needs you there. Do not be surprised if she enjoys going to the doctor. Foster children are often so needful of caring attention from others that they love a trip to the clinic.

EVALUATING A SICK CHILD

If a foster child says she is ill, it is important to find out what is truly going on with the child. Do not take her word that she is "burning up." If you use a regular fever thermometer, be sure to shake it down before using it. Any of the new devices for taking temperature are fine; just be sure and read the directions. Write down the temperature near the phone. Also, note any other symptoms, so that if you call the doctor, you will have the information handy.

If the child vomits or has diarrhea, try to take a look. If there is a rash, examine it. If the child's throat hurts, get a flashlight and look inside. You will be the one calling the doctor and you want to have as many facts as possible.

Very few childhood illnesses require urgent medical attention. You can usually wait an hour or two before calling the doctor. Try to calm the child and act as if you are not upset. Often, when the child calms down, the symptoms will improve.

NEED FOR EMERGENCY CARE

If a child has a very severe illness, he or she will usually appear quite ill. Of course, in this area, you may be handicapped by not knowing the child well. "Ian was about the twelfth foster child I had," said a foster mother. "One day he collapsed and I couldn't wake him. I finally picked him up and took him to the emergency room. He opened his eyes in the examining room and the doctor thought Ian had been faking. I guess I'll never know for sure. I didn't really regret overreacting, because he sure did look awfully sick."

The worst things children get are severe infections. In the case of meningitis, the child will have a high fever and will look quite ill. He may complain of headache and stiff neck. This is one situation where there should not be a delay in getting medical attention. A child with appendicitis also needs to go to the emergency room right away. The symptoms are pain in the right lower abdomen, vomiting, and fever. If you wait too long, the swollen appendix can burst and the treatment will be prolonged.

Certain breathing problems need a quick trip to the emergency room, and that includes asthma. The child with an asthma attack will usually sit on the edge of the bed and make a wheezing sound when breathing. There may be coughing, and the child may be quite distressed.

Two throat infections can cause trouble breathing. Epiglottitis is rare and occurs in older children. Symptoms are fever, difficulty in breathing, and difficulty in swallowing. Croup occurs in younger children and causes a barking cough and trouble with breathing. Call the doctor or clinic and use your judgment about going to the hospital.

If you go the emergency room, you may be there for a while. Take something to read or to do. Take all the papers for the child. After you get to the hospital, consider whether you need to call the caseworker or the child's birth parents.

GIVING MEDICATION

Remember that younger children may not be able to swallow pills. Most medication can be given in liquid form. The doctor needs to prescribe the medicine as a liquid. If you have pills and the child cannot swallow them, ask the pharmacist if the pills can be crushed.

Eye drops are frightening for some children. Have the child lie down and put the drops into the eye while it is closed. Then when she opens the eye, the drops will go in. Most creams and ointments need to be applied lightly and only to the area involved, but there are exceptions. Be sure to follow directions on the package.

Inhalers are commonly used for asthma. Ask the nurse in the clinic to explain the procedure and make sure you and the child understand. A machine called a nebulizer is sometimes used for asthma, especially in young children. The clinic nurse can teach you about it, and the person who delivers it from the company may also be helpful with instructions.

Make sure you know about the child's drug allergies. If he or she is allergic to any drugs, you must advise the doctor and the pharmacist. Also talk to the child and be sure the child knows about all allergies.

COLDS, COUGHS, AND SORE THROATS

Upper respiratory infections are seldom serious, but they can be troublesome. The viruses that cause most of these illnesses are passed easily from person to person. Careful handwashing may help prevent the spread. Most of these viruses have a short incubation period, so that others in the household may become ill within a week or two.

The common cold usually consists of stuffy nose, cough, slight fever, and sore throat. Very young children may have trouble sleeping. Older children may be irritable and uncomfortable. Coughing after a cold may continue for weeks. It is acceptable to use no medication for a cold. That saves money and the nuisance of getting children to take medicine. Antibiotics should not be used unless there is a complication. The usual cold remedies may provide a little comfort, but they do not shorten the course of a cold. Nose drops are not generally recommended.

Ear infections are a complication of a cold and may need antibiotics. Older children complain of earache, and younger children become quite fussy if their ears hurt. This is not an emergency, but if the earache does not get better in twenty-four hours, a doctor should be consulted. Hearing may be affected for a long time after an ear infection. However, the problem will usually resolve itself.

Sore throats that persist for more than twenty-four hours may be caused by the strep bacteria. A throat culture should be taken, and antibiotics may be administered. Infectious mononucleosis, which is sometimes called "mono," causes a persistent sore throat, droopiness, and swollen lymph glands. No treatment is needed, but if the illness persists the child may need a note from the doctor to stay out of school.

Croup is the childhood form of laryngitis. It causes a harsh "barking" cough, which is usually worse at night. Try taking the child into the bathroom and turning on the shower so that the room steams up. If that does not help, you may have to go to the hospital. Breathing treatments may be provided in the emergency room.

Nosebleeds can be a nuisance. Usually, they occur in the winter when the air is dry. Have the child pinch the nostril closed, gently, for five minutes. If it has not stopped after that, repeat the procedure. Check with the doctor if nosebleeds occur several times in a day. You may be told to gently put a little petroleum jelly inside the nose, for protection and lubrication. Keep the child's fingernails cut short, so that he does not cause the bleeding to start again.

STOMACHACHES, DIARRHEA, VOMITING, AND APPENDICITIS

Children often complain of stomachaches in the same way that adults complain of headaches. Foster children, who may be testing you to see if you love them, may complain persistently. A stomachache that goes on for many weeks and is not accompanied by weight loss seldom means very much. Pediatricians are used to this problem. The doctor will do some tests, examine the child, and will be reassuring. You can help by trying to distract the child and give her more positive ways to get your love and attention.

The sudden onset of a stomachache, of course, can signal illness. The first consideration is a stomach virus. These viruses often result in vomiting. Most children who vomit should be offered nothing by mouth for an hour or two. Older children may vomit a number of times without any serious danger. Young children and babies can become dehydrated and may need to be checked by a doctor. Diarrhea often comes after the vomiting has stopped and may last a day or two. You can switch to clear liquids or keep the child on a regular diet. Changing the diet does not seem to alter the course of this type of illness. Check with your doctor.

Appendicitis causes right lower abdominal pain. Often there are no bowel movements and there may be vomiting and fever. Sometimes the child cannot walk. Go to the emergency room and make sure that you have all the appropriate papers for the child with you. Take something to read and comforting items for the child. It may take a while for the child to be evaluated. Appendicitis is treated by surgery, and you will have to get consent for surgery from the child's guardian.

Urinary tract infections occur more often in girls than in boys. They often occur repeatedly, but you may not know this child's history. Tell the child that she may need to give the doctor a urine sample. If a child has a urinary infection, he or she may need special tests to make sure there is no problem in the bladder or kidneys. Symptoms of urinary tract infection are burning on urination, going to the bathroom frequently, and blood in the urine.

When a girl has lower abdominal pain or a boy has burning on urination, one needs to consider the possibility of a sexually transmitted disease. Also, pregnancy must be considered in all older girls. There is no age when one can guarantee that a foster child may not have had sexual contact. Try to be reasonable about this, but if you are concerned, be sure and talk to the doctor. If there is a sexually related problem, talk to the caseworker as soon as possible.

ASTHMA, BRONCHITIS, AND PNEUMONIA

All of these conditions cause coughing. The child with pneumonia or bronchitis may have a fever and not feel like eating. He or she may be quite droopy and may complain of pain in the chest or upper abdomen. Vomiting may occur. If the child seems quite ill, go to the doctor or emergency room.

If a child has symptoms of pneumonia or bronchitis and is not terribly ill, encourage the child to rest and drink lots of fluid. Talk to the doctor and describe the symptoms. Cough medicine is not necessary and neither is any other medicine unless the doctor recommends it. Antibiotics may be prescribed. You may need to visit the clinic with the child to get a note for the school.

As a child recovers from a respiratory illness, several days may pass before the appetite returns. You can pamper the child a little, with extra treats during that time. Coughing may continue for a very long time, but there is seldom any reason to be concerned about a child who coughs for several weeks.

Asthma attacks cause a child to wheeze. The child will sit on the edge of a bed and have obvious difficulty in breathing, especially breathing out. You will hear the sound of wheezing and if you look closely, you will see the neck and chest muscles working hard to move air in and out of the lungs. Try to have the child drink extra fluids and to relax. Use the child's inhalers or medication as prescribed. If an asthma attack persists and this child does not have an inhaler, go to the doctor or emergency room. Medication will be prescribed that can be used this time and in a future asthma attack.

ALLERGIC CONDITIONS

Certain childhood allergies are common. You may be told that your foster child is allergic to a food or to insects such as bees. Try to get the details of what has happened in the past. If there was a minor problem, you will probably not have an emergency. If the child had a serious allergic reaction in the past, you will have to be very careful. Often, there is no clear information. You will then have to assume that the allergic problem is serious.

Serious allergic reactions can occur due to certain foods, such as chocolate, peanuts, tomatoes, or fish. If the child is very young you will be responsible for her diet and you can monitor it. Be sure to read labels and try to cook most food from scratch. Older children will often eat away from home. The doctor or clinic may be helpful in teaching the child how to avoid foods that cause an allergic reaction.

With bee sting allergy, you may need a bee sting kit. This should be with the child whenever she is outdoors. If she is young, other caregivers at school and elsewhere need to be informed about emergency care. If she is an older child, she may be able to take care of herself. A bee sting kit comes with directions, but be sure to go over the details with the doctor. Treatment involves giving a shot of epinephrine when a bee sting has occurred. The medication can be life-saving and it has no particular risks.

Eczema is a scaly, itchy skin rash that is usually allergic. It is treated with oral antihistamines to decrease the itchiness and with hydrocortisone cream. Usually there is underlying dry skin, and lotion should be applied daily to those areas that are dry. Some children have involvement of large areas and the skin may ooze and become infected. Be sure the doctor is involved in such cases.

Hives are raised broad blotchy areas anywhere on the body that tend to come and go. They are allergic in origin, but the cause often is not known. Some people feel they can be caused by emotional stress. Antihistamines are used to relieve the itching.

CHICKENPOX AND OTHER CHILDHOOD ILLNESSES AND RASHES

Chickenpox is an illness that may be disappearing soon because of a vaccine. However, the vaccine is not yet widely used. Chickenpox starts out like a mild cold, then the characteristic rash appears. The first spots are usually on the trunk and may look like small blisters. As each blister begins to heal, a scab is formed. For several days there are blisters and scabs all over the body accompanied by fever and itching. The rash dries up in five or six days. A child with chickenpox should stay home from school for seven days.

The only other childhood rash with blisters is caused by contact with poison ivy, a plant that grows during the summer. It is not contagious and no treatment is needed.

Roseola is an illness of very young children. Typically, there is a high fever for several days followed by a rash, which is seen after the fever has gone. There is no danger with this illness. "Fifth disease" occurs in children of any age. It produces a "slapped face" appearance, where the face appears flushed, but there is often no illness or fever.

Scarlet fever is a strep infection in which a sore throat is accompanied by a reddish coloration of the skin and fever. Strep infections should be treated with antibiotics.

INFESTATIONS AND INFECTIONS THAT SPREAD

Head lice are mites that can live in the hair of the scalp. Sometimes, an actual small bug, or louse, may be seen jumping. More often the eggs of this bug, called nits, are attached to the hair shaft. The infestation is itchy and quite contagious. Children often get head lice at school. A foster child may bring head lice back from a visit to her birth home. Do not criticize the child for having lice. There are prescription and nonprescription treatments for head lice. Talk to the child's doctor. Plan to wash the child's bedding, stuffed animals, clothing, and coats. The eggs need to be pulled off by hand. They cannot be removed with a comb. A child cannot see the nits and so cannot remove them from his or her own hair.

Ringworm is a fungal infection of the skin, which takes the form of a circular, scaly area on the skin. Often there is only one spot or a few. It tends to be worst on the edges and healed in the center. It is not itchy. There is nonprescription treatment. You can try an antifungal cream from the pharmacy. Use extra precautions if the child is involved in sports, such as wrestling. Wash the clothes and bedclothes.

Impetigo is a skin rash caused by bacteria. There is usually a crusted rash around the nose and mouth. It may last several weeks until it is treated. It should be treated with antibiotic cream or oral antibiotics. The school nurse will send a child with impetigo home because it is contagious. You will need a note from the child's doctor before sending her back.

Scabies usually occurs in older children. It is caused by a mite that burrows into the skin. It produces small, red, itchy bumps, most often located in the groin, wrist, or fingers. Treatment is with a prescription lotion. You need to wash the bedclothes and the clothes. Check the rest of the family because it is quite contagious.

Pink eye (conjunctivitis) is an eye infection that spreads easily from child to child. It causes the white part of the eye to become pink or red, and there may be some crusting or itching. It is treated with antibiotic eye drops.

WOUNDS, SCRAPES, BITES, AND STITCHES

Many children have cuts and scrapes. Foster children are more susceptible, because their behavior is often more unpredictable. In most cases, take time to clean a wound and consider whether a trip to the hospital is necessary. Stitches are needed if a wound is gaping open. Sometimes staples are used or even glue. Make sure you take along the child's immunization records, as a tetanus shot may be required. Before leaving the emergency room, be sure you know how to protect the area and when to come back.

When there is an animal bite, such as from dogs or cats, wash the area with soap and water. If there is a puncture, take the child to the emergency room. Sometimes stitches are not used in bites in order to allow healing. The animal bite should be reported to the local authorities, as there is a question of rabies. Animals carry many bacteria, so antibiotics and a tetanus shot may be needed. In many areas, raccoons and other wild animals carry rabies. Your hospital emergency room should know how to handle this problem.

Any exposure to a bat should be considered an exposure to rabies. Go to the emergency room and discuss treatment with the doctor. It involves a series of shots, but the shots are not dangerous or painful.

BROKEN BONES

The most common fractures in children involve the collar bone, wrist, and elbow. If a child has had an injury, you should look at the area. Bruising or swelling is usually present if there has been a fracture. Also, there will be tenderness at the exact point of the fracture. Broken bones result from trauma. Child abuse may have caused such injuries in the past for your child. The emergency room staff may consider child abuse when any child is brought in with a fracture, so be prepared for possible questioning.

Fractures usually need to be treated in an emergency room. You may be able to wait a few hours until you can make arrangements. In most cases, the emergency room doctors will call an orthopedist to treat the child and you will have a return appointment to the orthopedist. Make sure you know all directions and precautions. Occasionally general anesthesia is necessary in order for the orthopedist to set the fracture or to put screws or other hardware in place. You will need the consent of the child's guardian for such surgery.

If your foster child has some kind of splint put on and is told to leave it on, you may find that the child takes it off after a few days. Foster children often also find ways to remove their own casts. Frustrated foster parents should call the orthopedist and inquire as to the need for having the cast replaced. The orthopedist should always be willing to put on another cast; he or she will probably lecture the child more firmly about the need for the cast. If it is a splint, and it is removable, you may find that the orthopedist is using it only for comfort, and the child may not need to wear it.

HEAD INJURY

If your foster child has a head injury, there are several possible reasons. Someone may have hit the child, there may have been a fall, or there may have been an automobile accident. Obviously, some head injuries are so severe that the child will need to go right to the emergency room.

In other cases, you will be the one to decide whether or not to go to the emergency room. You need to know if the child was unconscious, if there is any bleeding, and whether the child's vision is normal. If there was unconsciousness, even briefly, take the child to the hospital. If the child has blurry vision, take the child to the hospital. If there is bleeding, examine the wound. Remember that some small scalp wounds bleed a lot.

If you go to the hospital, take the child's medical cards and call the caseworker and biological family. Also take your knitting or a book to read. When you take a child who has had a head injury to the hospital, the doctor may need to do a CT scan in order to make sure there is no internal bleeding. That test takes some time, but is not painful. In most cases, the child will be sent back home. You may be asked to keep watch, for the first few hours, that he or she does not lose consciousness. Ask for specific directions about that and any other precautions.

If someone hit the child or the child was involved in a fight, school authorities or police may get involved. You may need to discuss the incident with the child after the medical emergency is over.

REASONS A CHILD MIGHT LIMP

When a child limps, there are a variety of possible causes. Sickle cell anemia can cause limping in an African-American child. A young child may fake limping, because he or she has watched another person limp. There may be a problem with the foot or ankle, such as a sliver or a blister.

If a child has had a fracture or sprain, you should see swelling or bruising in the area. However, a swollen knee or knee pain may not be very serious in children. A regular visit to the child's doctor may be appropriate, rather than a trip to the emergency room.

Hip problems in children can be difficult to diagnose. Several conditions occurring in children can cause limping and may cause pain in the upper leg or knee. The doctor will need to x-ray the knee and the hip. Generally, limping does not signal an emergency, but expert treatment is important.

CHILDHOOD CONDITIONS THAT REQUIRE SURGERY

If a foster child needs surgery, make sure that appropriate persons are available to sign consent. Often that means that the biological parent must be involved in the decision for surgery and must consent to it. If you have time to prepare the child for surgery, ask if the hospital lets children visit and get used to the place. Some hospitals have a program in which children are allowed to see and touch the equipment and meet the nurses.

Appendicitis is usually an emergency. It causes pain in the right lower side of the abdomen and occasionally elsewhere in the abdomen. Pain is usually accompanied by fever, vomiting, lack of appetite, and lack of bowel movements. Usually this happens without warning. The child has been feeling well, and the stomachache becomes severe over a few hours. If you suspect appendicitis, go to the emergency room. Surgeons want to remove an appendix if it is inflamed before it ruptures.

Hernias are common in boys of all ages. There is swelling of the scrotum, where the testicle is located. Any swelling in this area should be seen by a doctor, as emergency treatment may be necessary. A hernia is usually corrected by surgery. Although not a serious operation, it usually requires general anesthesia.

Children who have had frequent ear infections may have tubes put in their ears to allow air to flow through the eardrum and into the middle ear. This ventilation of the middle ear prevents ear infections in the future. The doctor may tell you not to let the child swim if there are tubes. Usually the tubes fall out in a few years.

Tonsils are still removed, although not nearly as commonly as in the past. If a child has quite large tonsils or has a history of recurring strep infections, tonsillectomy might be recommended. This is seldom done as an emergency.

Broken bones may or may not require surgery. Treatment of a fracture may be nothing more than putting on a cast. However, the orthopedist may need to "set" the fracture to straighten out the bone. If anesthesia or surgery is necessary, this would seem to indicate a serious break.

WHEN THERE IS BLEEDING—UNIVERSAL PRECAUTIONS

There are several viruses than can be carried in a person's blood, including hepatitis B and HIV. In these cases, the problem is contagious if there is a blood exposure. Universal precautions are used for all blood exposures, whether or not the person is known to carry any viruses.

Children may bleed from a nosebleed, from minor injuries on the playground, or from major injuries such as automobile accidents. If you are present when bleeding occurs, using universal precautions means that you should not touch the blood. Use gloves or some other type of protection. When you are finished tending the child, wash your hands thoroughly with soap and water. Dispose of all bloody material in a plastic bag, which has been tied shut.

In most cases, urine and stool do not carry infectious viruses. Changing diapers generally does not require gloves, but careful handwashing after diaper changes is recommended. There are no special precautions about diaper disposal.

Many diseases are spread by sexual contact. If a foster child shows interest in sexual activity, be sure to inform the child about the use of condoms to prevent the transmission of disease.

15

The Chronically Ill
Foster Child

Some foster children have a disability or a chronic illness. It takes a strong family to welcome such a child, as these children bring special challenges. Chronic diseases may affect various systems of the body and, consequently, many aspects of a child's life.

For a child with a disability, it can be distressing to need special tests and treatments. Many of these conditions last for a lifetime, and the child will continue to have problems and need care for many years. If a foster child's illness requires special treatment, it is important that the child learn to take care of his or her own needs. That means that the child needs to understand the disease, know where to go for help, and understand the treatment.

FOSTER HOMES FOR CHRONICALLY ILL CHILDREN

Some foster parents specialize in children with medical needs. Some have developed knowledge in a certain area from prior experiences. Other such foster parents are nurses or medical professionals with broad health care experience.

Some homes are not appropriate for foster children with chronic conditions. New foster families may not be ready for a child with an illness. Some foster families specifically ask for only healthy children. In some cases, a particular foster home might be unhealthy. Cigarette-smoking foster parents should not have an asthmatic foster child. A home without wheelchair access cannot have a child with spina bifida who uses a wheelchair.

Preparation for a child with a chronic condition would be helpful, but often that is not possible. Placement is usually quite sudden and the child may arrive without needed equipment or information. Sometimes the ideal foster home is not available and you may be asked to take a child with special medical needs. Such a child will be challenging, but taking the child will also be rewarding.

FOSTER CHILDREN WITH CHRONIC ILLNESS

It is difficult to learn to live with a chronic illness. If there is a strong family support system, a person will derive comfort from that. For foster children who do not have strong family support, learning to cope will be especially difficult. The illness, itself, may have contributed to the difficult home situation that resulted in placement. So guilt, anger, and frustration are common problems with the chronically ill foster child.

Compliance is a term for cooperation, and families that are troubled have often been noncompliant with medication and other treatments. Tests may not have been done and appointments may not have been kept. Consequently, the child may be functioning below his capabilities. You will have the opportunity to organize the child's care and to improve his level of functioning.

You may find that the child is embarrassed and ashamed of the illness. It is hard enough to be a foster child, but extra hard to be a sick foster child. The child may worry that you will not love him enough or care for him enough. Give him a chance to talk about this and try to find some way to comfort him. Point out the good things about him and try not to emphasize the negative things.

If your own child has a chronic condition, you can assume that you will be taking care of him until he has grown up. You might not feel a great need for him to understand the details of his condition. Foster children need to know everything about their own problems. At some point, they will move somewhere else and probably neither you nor their medical records will be with them. What is in the child's head will be extremely helpful and sometimes life saving.

GETTING STARTED WITH A FOSTER CHILD WITH SPECIAL HEALTH NEEDS

Consider the space you will allot the child. Can it handle the equipment she needs? Are there stairs, rugs, or furniture blocking the child from getting around? Does the bathroom need special equipment? Talk to the caseworker. There may be funding to pay for changes such as ramps and handrails. Pay special attention to issues of safety.

Is there a clinic where she has been going and where she is already known? Often foster parents have to do some detective work to find this information. Do you understand her medications and treatments? If not, call the clinic and tell personnel there your concerns. Find out when the child's next appointment is scheduled and what you should do in the meantime.

Has the child been cooperative in the past with her treatment? Does she take her own medication? Assume at first that you will need to monitor this. Chances are the child has been cutting corners and you need to know that.

Do you have a baby-sitter or family member who can care for the child when you go out? Your caseworker may be able to suggest a respite home if needed. How will you transport the child? Do you need handicapped license plates on your car?

Will the child need a special bus for transportaiton to school? What will the school nurse need? If the child takes medicine at school, the nurse will probably need a separate prescription and a pharmacy-labeled container.

HELPING A FOSTER CHILD WITH SPECIAL HEALTH CONCERNS

Foster children who are healthy often are embarrassed about being in foster care. They feel that everyone is talking about them and that no one likes them. Having a medical condition makes all that worse. Just as you need to build on the strengths of all foster children, you should take special care to make such a child comfortable. Be very careful what you say to and about her.

Do as much as you can to relieve the physical symptoms. At the clinic, you may have to be a strong advocate to get medications changed or tests done. If you feel the child is not doing well, tell the doctor. After you are certain that all is being done that can be done, help the child to learn to adjust to the symptoms and problems that remain. Try not to let the child dwell on her problems. Tell her that you will listen to her, but you would rather talk about something else. The clinic may know of a support group of parents or children with a similar condition. That would be very helpful for a foster parent and a foster child as they adjust together to the problems of the illness.

If there are things that you and the child can do to slow the progress of the illness, make sure she understands these things and help her cooperate. If she needs a special diet, be as helpful as you can about providing it. If exercise is important, exercise with her. If she needs to monitor blood sugar levels, watch while she does this.

If your foster child needs tests or procedures that are uncomfortable, try very hard to be with her during that time. This is the time a child most needs her mother or father and you are the substitute parent. Your knowledge will also help when the next episode is coming up. You and the child may figure out ways to make it more tolerable.

Professionals sometimes react with annoyance at foster children. Treatment plans may not have been followed and past information may not be available. Also, the child represents a problem that people often are not comfortable with—that is, the problem of troubled families. If a professional reacts to your foster child with displeasure, try to be a peacemaker. Speak up for the child and tell the professional that you and the child are doing fine now.

As the child grows older, she needs to learn to be comfortable with professionals who are taking care of her. She needs to speak up, to ask questions, to help make appointments, and to follow up on recommendations. If the biological family has been difficult in the past, it is even more important to teach her to interact well with professionals.

HIGH-TECH NEWBORN CARE

Hospital care of a sick newborn has become so successful that many babies who were born weighing less than a pound now survive. Organs may have been too immature to function and machines were used to breathe for the baby and provide nutrition. Gradually, as the baby grew older, systems began to function. A baby may be ready to go home and still need special assistance and protection.

Premature birth is common for women in poverty, women on drugs, and women who have not had prenatal care. Many such mothers are not fit to take their children home and the babies will enter the foster care system. This may be a temporary placement, or it may be the beginning of a permanent plan for adoption.

If you are willing to take a newborn foster child with continuing needs, you should get assistance from several sources. Nursing care will be available and medical care and equipment will be provided. Plan to ask questions of every professional involved with the child so that you can learn as much as possible.

A high-needs baby not only requires technical assistance, but also needs lots of love. Hold the baby as much as you can and talk and sing to her. If appropriate, try to get the biological mother involved in the baby's care. Many foster parents learn to love such a baby and then have difficulty giving the child up. Chances are that the child will either return to the biological mother or be adopted by another family member. It is actually unusual that the foster parents can adopt such a child.

ASTHMA

Asthma is increasingly common, and the disease seems to occur often in impoverished homes and in slums. Although it is quite rare to die of asthma, there are more such deaths now than in the past. During an asthma attack, the small airways in the chest are constricted or tight. People often describe a feeling of tightness, and wheezing, or noisy breathing, is a classic symptom. Asthmatics feel short of breath when they are having an attack, but between attacks they generally feel fine. Most asthma in children is caused by allergy. Common causes are cigarette smoke, pets (particularly cats), pollen, and dust. Some children wheeze when they exercise.

Treatment is with bronchodilators, or medicines that open up the airways, and most are given by inhaler. Sometimes inhaled drugs are taken several times a day on a regular basis. With mild asthma, the inhaler is usually only used when needed. Younger children may use a machine (nebulizer) instead of an inhaler because they cannot handle an inhaler. Older children who have severe forms of asthma also may use a nebulizer.

If a child has an asthma attack, try using the inhaler and then have her lie down. Sit with her and try to distract her. See if she calms down and breathing gets easier. If the child does not get better, you will have to go to a clinic or emergency room. There the child will be given medication and may get blood tests and a chest X ray. Occasionally, hospitalization is necessary.

JUVENILE RHEUMATOID ARTHRITIS

In general, this is the only form of arthritis that occurs in children. It can involve various joints of the body, especially the joints of the hands. A child with rheumatoid arthritis may appear quite ill when the disease is active. He or she may have a fever and not be able to move well. Because the disease causes pain in the joints and it hurts to move, a child with arthritis may stay so still that the joints and limbs actually stiffen up. So the child needs to be encouraged to move about whenever possible. Special tests are needed to be sure that the condition is rheumatoid arthritis. Rarely, other types of arthritis are identified and the treatment for these conditions would be quite different.

Medication for rheumatoid arthritis can be as simple as aspirin, although aspirin should only be used under medical supervision. Other drugs are useful and physical therapy may be an important part of treatment. This disease can go away as the child grows up, or it may be present for a lifetime. Specialists need to be involved when the disease is active to try to avoid permanent damage.

If special equipment is needed for a child with rheumatoid arthritis, it will be available through the doctor's office or the therapist. Such a child may need special devices to learn to feed herself if the arms are affected. She may need a wheelchair if the legs are involved.

CONGENITAL HEART DISEASE

Some congenital heart defects are mild and correction is not necessary. Other defects may have been completely corrected by the time you get a child. In either of these cases you will probably need to go to a special clinic once a year, and you may have to give the child an antibiotic before dental work. If you do not have information on a child's condition, try calling the nearest university with a pediatric cardiology clinic to see if the child is registered there.

A child may come to you with a severe heart defect that is not fully corrected. In most cases, this child will have had some testing already. Again, you need to contact the clinic and find out when the next appointment is scheduled. Confirm any medications and any special precautions. Make sure that the child can be fully active. If surgery is in the child's future, you usually have a lot of time to get ready. There is paperwork and the child needs to be prepared. The birth family and caseworker will probably be involved.

Common moderately severe defects are atrial septal defect, ventricular septal defect, coarctation of the aorta, and patent ductus arteriosus. Severe defects are tetralogy of Fallot, transposition of the great arteries, and hypoplastic left heart. All are treated with surgery, and some children need more than one operation.

Children with congenital heart defects may have other problems, such as Down's syndrome, but most often they are normal in other ways. Serious cardiac defects are often accompanied by learning problems.

CYSTIC FIBROSIS

This severe lung disease in children is inherited. Basically, there are two problems. One problem is that the ducts in the pancreas are plugged and certain pancreatic enzymes are not produced. The enzymes can be given in pill form and that prevents diarrhea and weight loss due to malnutrition.

The lung problem is more difficult to treat. A child with cystic fibrosis has thick secretions in the lungs. At first, such children have occasional lung infections, such as pneumonia or bronchitis. These infections heal slowly, because coughing cannot bring up the sticky secretions. Eventually, lung infections become severe. Persons with this condition usually die of respiratory failure around the age of thirty, unless they have a lung transplant.

The disease occurs equally in boys and girls and it is inherited from both parents, who are usually carriers of the cystic fibrosis gene. The child may have a brother or sister with the disease. It becomes clear to most of these children at quite a young age that they have a fatal disease.

Children with cystic fibrosis are treated with strong antibiotics for long periods of time. They may need special treatments for their breathing, and they need to be followed by a pediatric pulmonary specialist. Treatment is very important so that these children can continue to be active in school and in the neighborhood. Everyone will need to make special arrangements for periods of illness and for hospitalizations.

DIABETES

Unlike adults with diabetes, children almost always need to take insulin. Insulin is given by injection, and older children usually give their own injections. Injections may be given several times a day, but usually twice is adequate. Two kinds of insulin are often mixed in the syringe.

Usually blood sugar readings are taken once or twice a day. This involves a piece of equipment that is fairly simple to operate. There is a finger stick and a drop of blood. Diabetic children need to record their blood sugars and insulin dosages in a logbook.

Diet is not usually terribly strict, but diabetic children need to eat a sensible diet on a reasonable schedule. Insulin lowers blood sugar and eating raises blood sugar. Diabetics cannot delay meals or their insulin will cause low blood sugar. Exercise is important and should also occur at the same time each day. Exercise lowers the blood sugar, as it uses energy. Late afternoon is a time when many diabetics have trouble with low blood sugar, also called hypoglycemia. They may become silly or angry or droopy. It is important for them to get milk or orange juice at that time to build up their blood sugar.

A doctor needs to be in close communication with the family. Insulin dosages may change on a day-to-day basis so as to keep the child's blood sugar level at a near-normal reading. Diabetic foster children will need to be closely monitored by foster parents at the beginning. As children grow older, they take more responsibility for giving insulin, testing blood sugar, and managing their lifestyle.

Diabetic children are often placed in a home with a nurse or with a diabetic family member. This makes managing the disease much easier. If the child is confused about the disease or is uncooperative, try to ease these problems during the stay in your home. That will be helpful to the child in the next placement or upon returning to the birth home. Teach the child to keep a record of blood sugar levels, insulin dosage, doctor's appointments, hypoglycemic reactions, and other incidents.

The long-term effects of diabetes usually do not occur during childhood. Diabetic women may have difficult pregnancies. Infants of diabetic mothers may be extra large or may be deformed in some way. Blindness, kidney failure, and heart disease are common problems that occur in adults who have been diabetic for many years. Keeping blood sugar levels near normal helps delay these long-term complications.

HEADACHES

Migraine headaches usually begin in the early teenage years. A migraine is a throbbing one-sided headache. It may be preceded by a sense of flashing lights or some other visual abnormality. The headache lasts from several hours to all day and may involve vomiting. The person generally falls asleep at the end. During a migraine most people want darkness and quiet. Certain things may seem to cause headaches, such as stress, sleeping late, or certain foods.

There is treatment for migraine. The first thing to do is try a mild pain reliever and rest. If the problem persists, see the doctor. Stronger pain medicines may be used. Also medication may be tried preventively. That is often difficult, as headaches do not occur very often and most children do not like taking medicine.

Children sometimes have other types of headaches. Sinus infections or a bad cold can cause headaches. Headaches may be symptoms of brain tumors or brain infections. Sometimes a CT scan may be ordered to make sure there is no abnormality of the brain. A CT scan is not painful, but it requires being still for a period of time. Some young children may need to be sedated.

LEAD POISONING

This is a problem in old housing or impoverished neighborhoods. The paint used in old houses had lead in it and it may still be there, buried under more recent layers of paint. If paint starts to peel off the walls, doors, windows, radiators, or porches, the child may eat the chips of paint and lead will build up in the body. High lead levels cause brain damage. Even slight elevations in lead level can affect intelligence.

All young children should be screened for lead poisoning at around one year of age. If the level is normal, most children need no more testing. Older foster children may have lived in various environments and they may not have been tested at the age of one year. When the doctor asks about lead poisoning and the child is new to you, suggest that a test be done.

If lead level is elevated, the first step is to remove the lead hazard from a child's environment. Testing of the home should be followed with repair if lead is present. The parents need to wet mop the floor and clean radiators and windowsills. If lead levels are very high, treatment of the child may be necessary. Treatment usually requires hospitalization.

LEUKEMIA AND CHILDHOOD CANCERS

Childhood cancers are not the same as adult cancers. They are, fortunately, quite rare. In many cases, treatment is fairly successful, perhaps more so than in adult cancers. However, the treatment is frightening for a child. A foster child might come to you having been successfully treated for cancer. Or a child may be in the midst of treatment, which can go on for years. Cancer might develop while a child is in your care.

Leukemia, the most common childhood cancer, it is an overproduction of white blood cells. It usually begins when a child is between two and five years old. Early signs are bruising, weight loss, and tiredness. A blood test usually identifies the disease, but a bone marrow test is necessary to determine exactly what kind of leukemia it is and how it should be treated. Over half of these children now survive and are considered cured.

Brain tumors in children cause headache and vomiting. Diagnosis is by CT scan. Some brain tumors can be removed successfully. Others end in death. Two other childhood cancers are Wilms' tumor, which is a cancer of the kidney, and retinoblastoma, which is a cancer of the eye. Both can be treated successfully in many cases, but the treatment is difficult.

SEIZURES

Epilepsy is a condition of recurring seizures. An epileptic child may be otherwise normal; however, epilepsy may occur in a child who is retarded or has other signs of brain damage. Children who have been abused sometimes have had head injury and may have seizures because of that.

A seizure is a short period of unconsciousness, and there may be some jerking of the arms and legs. A "grand mal" seizure starts suddenly and the person falls to the ground. There may be a short period of not breathing, when the child is quite stiff. Then the jerking begins and lasts two to three minutes. Other types of seizures may be quite short and involve only some mental confusion. The person may not fall to the ground or have any jerking.

The most important thing to remember, in caring for a child with seizures, is to give the child's medicine on a regular schedule. In this situation a missed pill, or even a late pill, may cause serious problems. Always watch a foster child taking seizure medicine. The child may be tempted to cheat and then a seizure will result. Make sure you know of a doctor's office or clinic where you can call someone twenty-four hours a day. Seizure medications need to be carefully balanced. Too much medication can cause lethargy and droopiness. If there is too little medication, there will be seizures. Most doctors test blood levels at least twice a year.

If a seizure occurs, have the child lie down, loosen the clothes, and watch carefully. If it is the first seizure, you should call for help, and if it goes on for twenty minutes, you should call an ambulance. Most seizures do stop on their own, and after you get to know a child and the pattern of seizures, you will not need to worry so much. It is extremely important to be helpful and comforting when the child begins to wake up. The child may be confused and frightened.

Make sure the child wears an identification bracelet with information about the seizure disorder. Be sure the school knows what to do. The child should never be allowed to swim alone, so you must consider this if you, or a neighbor, have a pool. If the child is older, there will be special considerations about driving, about getting pregnant, and about drinking alcohol. Be sure to talk to the doctor about these things and be sure the child is listening.

The nature of foster care is that the child will not be with you in the future. The child needs to be fully informed of her own health care needs, so that she can take care of herself if she returns home or goes into another placement. Teach the child to keep a record of visits to the doctor, medications, seizures, and any other problems.

SICKLE CELL ANEMIA AND OTHER BLOOD DISEASES

Sickle cell anemia is inherited and usually occurs in African Americans. It comes from both of the child's parents. The disease causes a persistent anemia and episodes of severe pain in the abdomen, arms, or legs. Such an episode is called a "pain crisis."

Children with sickle cell disease are hospitalized frequently and followed closely by a doctor, usually a pediatric hematologist. As yet, there is no treatment that will result in a cure, but new treatments are being tested, and your foster child may be involved in these treatments. Life expectancy is shortened. As these persons become adults, they will have a high likelihood of serious medical problems, such as heart attacks and strokes.

Hemophilia is a condition that, like sickle cell anemia, requires close monitoring by a pediatric hematologist. This is a bleeding disorder and is treated by giving an intravenous transfusion of a substance called factor VIII. Persons with hemophilia cannot produce their own factor VIII. Without factor VIII, a person would bleed whenever there was a cut or an injury.

With these and other genetic conditions, it is extremely important that children understand the reasons for treatment, the possibilities of problems in the future, and ways to stay well. It is also important that older children understand the genetic aspects. They need to know how this disease fits in with their own birth families. Also, they need to understand it, so that there will be no unnecessary risk for future children.

CROHN'S DISEASE

Crohn's disease and several other diseases of the gastrointestinal tract are called "inflammatory bowel diseases." Symptoms include diarrhea, weight loss, and fatigue. These are life-long conditions. Symptoms are absent at times and then return unpredictably. Treatment may be quite complex.

For all of these diseases, diarrhea and fatigue affect the lifestyle. Diet may be important. Special ways to make sure nutrition is maintained may involve feeding tubes or intravenous feedings. Surgery may be done to remove the inflamed part of the bowel. Such surgery does not usually result in a cure, but may improve the symptoms.

A child who has had surgery for inflammatory bowel disease may have a colostomy or an ileostomy. This is an opening that the surgeon has created in the wall of the abdomen. The patient keeps a plastic bag over the opening and stool is collected in the bag. Such a "stoma" may be temporary or permanent.

If a child has a disabling chronic condition, such as Crohn's disease, life will be difficult. If the child is also in foster care, the situation may cause many dilemmas. The child may be irritable, frustrated, or uncooperative. As with any chronic illness, you must continue to be as optimistic as possible. Keep a cheerful outlook to encourage the child to feel better about himself.

CEREBRAL PALSY

Cerebral palsy is caused by brain damage and is present at birth or appears within the first few years of life. It may not be noticed until the child is a toddler and the characteristic tightness appears. Limbs that are involved are weak and tend to be held in a stiff, curled fashion. If one or both legs are involved, the child will have a limp or may not walk at all. If an arm is involved, or both arms, there will be difficulty with daily activities. With mild cerebral palsy, the children often have normal intelligence. However, with the more severe forms there is usually some mental retardation.

Some children with cerebral palsy have trouble talking and will need the help of a speech therapist. Some cannot walk well and will need a physical therapist. Generally cerebral palsy does not get more or less severe over time. In other words, if a child is disabled with cerebral palsy, that child will continue to have the same disability throughout life. Many persons learn to overcome their handicaps with special equipment and special help. Your goal, with a child such as this, will be to encourage the child to be as independent as possible.

FOSTER CHILD IN A WHEELCHAIR

The reasons a child might need a wheelchair include cerebral palsy, spina bifida, muscular dystrophy, and severe mental retardation. Wheelchairs are usually ordered by a physical therapist. Frequent repairs may be necessary. A child will need a new wheelchair every year or so, as he or she grows.

A young child in a wheelchair is not much different from a regular toddler. Older children have problems of accessibility and have difficulty becoming independent. They may need help getting in and out of a car and they may have problems with toileting. The school may need to make special arrangements for a child in a wheelchair.

If it appears that the child will be with you for a while, explore the possibility of adapting your home to meet his needs. This may involve a ramp for getting outside, the lowering of faucets and the widening of doors.

Familiarize yourself with access in the community. Be an advocate for the child for facilities to become more accessible at school or in public places. You may have an agency in the community whose mission is to help disabled persons, and they can advise you and the child about facilities and programs that are available. Explore the possibility of wheelchair sports, if appropriate.

SPINA BIFIDA

This is a condition, present at birth, involving permanent damage to the spinal cord, usually in the low back. The area is exposed at birth, but usually there will have been a surgical repair soon after birth during which the surgeon will have covered the area with skin.

The child will have paralysis that involves only the legs, not the arms. The legs will be partially or completely paralyzed. The child will often also have problems with bowel and bladder. Toilet training will usually not be started until about the age of five. At that time, most children with spina bifida can be dry most of the time. However, some need to continue to catheterize themselves or use diapers part of the time.

Children with spina bifida often also have hydrocephalus, a build-up of excessive fluid in the brain, and the head actually may be overlarge. Treatment is to insert a shunt, draining the fluid from the brain to the belly. The shunt is not visible, but it often can be felt in a vein in the neck.

A child with spina bifida has paralysis of the legs, but also has no feeling in the lower body. For that reason, the child is prone to getting a bedsore if she does not move about in her wheelchair. She needs to learn to raise herself up in the chair by her arms, several times an hour during the day. If the child becomes overweight or is frequently wet, the likelihood of developing a bedsore will increase.

Usually there is a spina bifida clinic for these children, and your foster child may already have been seen there. If not, try to get the child enrolled. The clinic has professionals who can help with the various problems that accompany spina bifida.

MUSCULAR DYSTROPHY

This is an inherited disease, which is a result of the mother's abnormal genetic pattern, not the father's. It only occurs in boys. The child looks normal until about the age of two, when he should start to run and to climb stairs. He does not seem to progress in these areas, and gradually the parents note a waddling gait and other signs of muscle weakness. A diagnosis is usually made by a biopsy of the muscles of the leg.

Boys with muscular dystrophy begin to get weaker by the time they start school. They cannot get up off the floor or climb stairs. They begin to fall more often. By the age of ten, they are often using braces, and in adolescence, they are using a wheelchair. As the disease worsens, their arms also weaken, and eventually they may require an electric wheelchair. By the late teenage years, they begin to have pneumonia and trouble with breathing because the muscles of the chest become weak. Death usually occurs by about age twenty.

No treatment is helpful in terms of stopping the progression of the disease. Therapists prescribe exercises that help the child function longer. If it is hard to get cooperation with a child about exercises, consider joining a gym where he can get regular exercise in a more normal environment.

The disease is occasionally present in a brother. The biological mother of a son with muscular dystrophy should know that, if she becomes pregnant, she risks having another child with the disease.

AUTISM

Autism causes problems with language and lack of ability to interact socially. An autistic child has probably had the problem since early in life. The cause of autism is not known. In the past, it was thought to be caused by poor parenting. Now it is thought to be due to abnormal brain chemistry and to genetic factors.

Autism causes limitation in language development. Although language may develop, it will be unusual. The child may sing, recite television commercials, learn the alphabet, and yet not be able to have a meaningful conversation. One feature of autism is the tendency for a child to repeat questions back to you, rather than answer them.

These children seem remote and unsociable. They are relatively uninterested in other people, yet may be fascinated with objects, such as vacuum cleaners. Activities are quite repetitive and, as with the language problem, play is abnormal. Autistic children do not play with others well and they do not play alone in a meaningful way.

Autistic children are remote, distant, uninterested in others, and delayed in speech development. If your foster child is over the age of two and has some of these features, he or she might be diagnosed with the condition. Some children are not severely impaired, yet they have "autistic tendencies." Such a child may be quite similar to children with attachment problems or to children who have been abused.

There is no specific treatment for autism. No medication has proved useful, and no educational approach seems to help dramatically. Many persons with mild autism are able to function in life with only minor difficulties. Severely autistic children will probably be programmed in school along with mentally retarded children in special classrooms.

MENTAL RETARDATION

At an early age, a child who is retarded may have delays in development. That means that walking may not occur by fifteen months, as it does in normal children. Language may be more limited than with other children of the same age, as in a three-year-old who speaks only single words.

Mild forms of mental retardation are sometimes not noticed until a child starts school. A child may be unable to learn letters or numbers, unable to learn to write his or her name. The child may be asked to repeat kindergarten or first grade.

If you feel that a foster child is not doing as well in school as she should, arrange for testing. Intelligence testing may determine that the child is not retarded, in which case you will need to help her to catch up and keep up. If intelligence testing indicates that the child is retarded, you need to look for a possible cause.

Make an appointment to see the child's doctor. Ask that the child be checked for lead poisoning, thyroid problems, or anemia. Make sure the child is not taking any medication that might lead to mental confusion. There are several conditions that cause mental retardation, the most common being Down's syndrome (see page 185). In these cases, the developmental delays are usually fairly severe. The doctor should be able to arrange for testing if a medical condition is suspected. The doctor should also check the child's vision and hearing.

In many cases, foster children have delays in development due to getting a difficult start in life. The child may have been abused or neglected. Children who have been hungry, who have had untreated infections, or who are anxious about the future may have developmental delays. If problems such as these have caused the child's delays, he or she may be able to improve and eventually be normal.

A child who is delayed in language or physical development qualifies for various programs. Educational approaches may be individually designed for the child. In most areas, schooling for retarded persons begins at age three and continues to the age of twenty-one. Therapy may be available, either physical therapy to improve physical development or speech therapy to improve language, or both. Try to take advantage of all services that are available for the foster child.

With a retarded foster child, some arrangements will probably have to be made for living as an adult. Some older retarded individuals live in family care, which is similar to foster care.

SCHIZOPHRENIA

Schizophrenia is an adult psychiatric condition that may start in the teenage years. It tends to run in families. As children, these persons may have had poor social adjustment and clumsiness. As a teen, the child will begin to withdraw. The later stages of schizophrenia involve hallucinations, which means hearing voices that are not there.

Schizophrenic patients used to be institutionalized after diagnosis, often for the rest of their lives. Now that is not necessary, because medication can be quite effective. However, most schizophrenic patients need a lifetime of supervision. They need to be encouraged to take their medication, and they often need guidance in the various ways an adult needs to function.

DOWN'S SYNDROME

Down's syndrome is a genetic defect that is apparent at birth. The baby is somewhat floppy, and there are characteristic features of the face and hands. Down's syndrome children are usually easy to manage as infants. They are often rather placid. Development will be delayed once the child is old enough to walk and talk.

A Down's syndrome child will qualify for various programs for handicapped babies and other services from the time he or she is born. Special school will probably begin at three years of age. Some Down's syndrome children can function in elementary school in a regular classroom. Most do not, and are placed in a special education setting.

Some Down's syndrome children have congenital heart disease and need surgery to correct it. Some defects are quite severe and some are actually fatal. Many of these children need glasses and some are visually impaired, even with glasses. Having the child's eyes tested may be difficult for younger children, because they cannot cooperate with the testing. Hearing may also be abnormal.

Raising a Down's syndrome child is difficult for any parent, but it is especially challenging for a substitute parent. At any age, the child will not be able to tell you much about his history and will not be able to understand the details of what you are trying to ask or tell him. It will require extra patience to work with this child, but the rewards are great. Most Down's syndrome people are friendly and calm and pleasant family members. School will generally continue past the age of eighteen. Planning for this child, as he becomes an adult, will be very important.

HIV/AIDS

Children may get the HIV virus from their mothers at birth. Many HIV-positive children end up being in foster care because their mothers are unable to care for them. In general, foster parents will be told if a child coming to them is HIV-positive. Most children who are HIV-positive need treatment in a specialized clinic. If you suspect HIV in a foster child and do not know the test results, ask the caseworker or the doctor. You need to know.

Treatment is quite specialized. It involves some medication against the virus itself and some drugs to prevent other infections.

If a young HIV-positive child is in your home, you will be concerned about possible transmission. The virus is carried in the child's blood and will only be spread if the child bleeds. Even then, it must enter someone else's blood stream to be transmitted. So it is extremely unlikely that this will happen. You need to be careful whenever any child is bleeding, because you do not know what viruses might be in the blood. Use care and wash your hands. There are almost no examples of a family caregiver getting HIV from an HIV-positive person or child.

In an older HIV-positive child there are problems regarding self-care and regarding sexual behavior. The child needs to talk to a counselor in the HIV clinic about these things and so do you. What if he has a nosebleed in school? You and the child need to have a plan about these matters.

Confidentiality is important. The doctor and the school nurse and the caseworker are the only people that must know that a foster child is HIV-positive. However, the actual fact is that others will probably find out.

HOSPITALIZATION OF A FOSTER CHILD

In most cases, a foster parent cannot legally give permission for hospitalization or for surgery. For a child who has a chronic illness, you will have to work this out in advance. You must know how to reach the biological parents and the caseworkers at all times.

It is a good policy to try to have someone stay with a child who is hospitalized. If this is not possible, try to have someone visit often. Children get better care if there is a family member present, keeping an eye on things. It indicates that someone cares about the child.

Hospital procedures may be quite frightening for a child. Try to get as much advance information as you can so that you can help explain what is happening. Remember to talk things through with the child. If you just assume that she is handling things well, you might be surprised to learn how nervous and worried she really is.

A foster child who goes into the hospital may be worried that she will not go back home to you. Talk about future plans following the hospitalization. Make sure the child knows that you are planning to have her return to you.

DEATH OF A FOSTER CHILD

All of the diseases described in this chapter can be life-threatening. Children do die. Most likely death will not be sudden, and you and the child will have many months or years to deal with the issue of dying before it actually happens.

Most doctors now feel that anyone who has a fatal disease deserves to know the truth about that disease. At the same time, it is always appropriate to hold out hope to a child. For dying children, there are periods when they realize they will die soon and other periods when they deny it, even to themselves. As a caregiver, you will have the same swings from denial to acceptance and back.

With a terminally ill child you need all the supports of the community. You need a caring and knowledgeable physician, an attentive spouse and family, close access to clergy, and availability of volunteers and professionals for caregiving. You should not hesitate to ask for all of these for a terminally ill foster child. Be very careful to involve the biological parents and extended family members whenever possible.

CARDIOPULMONARY RESUSCITATION

Children seldom have heart attacks or heart rhythm disturbances, which are the reasons most adults have cardiac arrests. Yet, there are several situations when children may have cardiac arrest and a foster parent should be prepared. Every community provides inexpensive courses in CPR (cardiopulmonary resuscitation). Make sure you take the part of the course that covers CPR in children. To remain certified you may need to take the course every year or two years.

Very young babies may have apnea monitors and other specialized equipment because of breathing problems. Foster parents need to be CPR-certified if they take such a baby into their home. Apnea means absence of breathing, so if the monitor alarm goes off, the baby may have stopped breathing and CPR will be necessary.

Any foster family who has a swimming pool should take very special precautions regarding pool safety. However, tragedies may occur even with the best of intentions. CPR in a child who has almost drowned (called "near-drowning") may be very effective. Children do have the ability to recover from such a life-threatening event.

Other times when a child might need CPR seem like remote possibilities for most foster parents. Drug or alcohol overdose can occur with older children. Tragedy might be prevented by the presence of a person trained in resuscitation. Also, in sports settings where older children are under great stress, cardiac arrest can occur, though rarely.

A foster parent would not be wasting time learning CPR. Cardiac arrest may occur unexpectedly in the community or at the site of an automobile accident. The opportunity to step in and try to save a life is very satisfying.

16

Particular Concerns of Foster Parents

Foster parents have certain concerns that they often express in interviews and conversations. A major concern is that foster parents are not always treated with respect. Most foster parents have experience and love to offer to the children, yet the public remains suspicious of their motivations. Adoption, attachment, and allegations are frequent themes in discussions with foster parents. This chapter addresses the particular issues that foster parents are struggling with and offers some suggestions, many from other foster parents.

Foster parents tend to say that their opinions are ignored when it comes to deciding on the children's futures. In foster care the judges makes decisions about the children. If judges listened to all sides of each issue and thought things through carefully, foster parents might be happier. However, the judges often do not seem thoughtful, nor do they seem fair.

ADOPTING FOSTER CHILDREN

I've had Amy since she was a baby and now she's four. I know that parental termination is coming up and I want to adopt her. I've heard that the biological grandmother wants to adopt her, and that's where she'll probably go. I don't think it's fair. What can I do?

Sometimes, even though it should not be this way, people go into foster care because they want to adopt a child. If that was actually your motive, there will be much heartache ahead. As one foster parent said, "If adoption is what you really want to do, get out of foster care and consider foreign adoption."

Foster parents develop a natural attachment to a child they take care of and sometimes it seems appropriate to try to adopt the child when he or she becomes available. Unfortunately, the court may not allow this. One reason is that, if a biological family member wants the child, the judge must place that child with kin.

A second reason you may not be able to adopt a foster child is the need to place siblings together in one adoptive home. The court is expected to try to do that, and the judge will need to determine the best home for all of the children.

A third problem is the slow pace of the court system. There has been an effort to speed up the process of permanent placement of foster children, but, currently, even after termination of parental rights, it takes two-to-three years for adoption to be finalized.

The most common reason for the long wait for adoption is that the biological parents have stayed in the picture and termination has been delayed. If you are a foster parent who did start taking foster children for the "right" reason, to give the child some respite and then reunite the family, you should not be secretly hoping to adopt the child. Such an internal conflict will cause many problems. You cannot have it both ways, wishing to reunite and wishing to adopt.

ATTACHMENT PROBLEMS

DeeDee had an attachment problem. She had been abused until she was a year and a half. When she came to me, she couldn't walk or talk, didn't look at me, didn't smile. Now she's started school and she just doesn't seem to pay any attention to myself or to anyone else. The teacher is annoyed with her and so am I. I've done so much for this child.

When foster parents refer to attachment problems, they are usually talking about a child who did not form a good relationship with the biological mother and now does not seem to be forming relationships with anyone else. She is not affectionate, and when she gets into trouble, she does not seem to mind the punishment. Most foster parents are warm and affectionate people. They are surprised and disappointed when a foster child is unresponsive to them. Relatives are also disappointed and the caseworker is discouraged. Medication does not help and behavior plans are not effective.

This issue takes on great significance with many foster parents. Foster parents become quite vocal and angry about such a child, who gives so little back to them. The anger of these foster parents is partly caused by their own inappropriate expectations. Are you taking foster children for the "wrong" reasons? If, rather than reunification of a family, you are looking for a little child who will give you a lot of satisfaction, then you may be quite disappointed.

HIDDEN REASONS FOR BECOMING FOSTER PARENTS

My husband and I have had thirty-seven different foster children under our roof, at some time over the past eighteen years. I think we helped a lot of those kids grow up to be stronger and more successful. I don't see why these other foster parents complain all the time. They're just wasting their time and energy.

Foster parents have all taken a training course and all have had foster care explained. They should understand that foster care is temporary placement of a troubled child from a troubled family, and reunification of the biological family is usually the goal. This explanation is widely agreed upon by child care experts, judges, and the federal government. Nevertheless, many foster parents have secret reasons for taking foster children, besides reunification with the biological families. You may or may not realize that you have these secret desires.

Many foster parents secretly want a child to love them, a child to show off to their relatives, a child who will do what they tell them, a child to help around the house, or a child to adopt. The worst problems occur when a foster parent has a secret sexual interest in the child. People become angry and frustrated when these secret desires are not fulfilled.

If you have not yet started in foster care, consider these issues. If you have difficulty accepting the current definition of foster care and the idea of reuniting biological families, do not go into foster care. If, more than anything, you want to adopt a child, consider adopting an older child who is available or a foreign adoption.

CASEWORKER PROBLEMS

My caseworker has been in the business a long time. She doesn't have any children herself. She doesn't seem to like the kids and she doesn't seem to like me. I think our relationship should be better, because we're usually sort of hostile and that can't be good for the kids.

You may be right about this professional. He or she may be sick of the work and frustrated by the biological families and some of the other foster families. The caseworker may not have let herself learn about you, and as you always feel a little angry, you are probably not communicating very well with her.

Ask the caseworker to stop by when there are no children around, then fix coffee and sit down. Ask her how things are going and let her talk. Tell her that you realize the job is hard and try to think of something specific to praise her about. Ask about some of her success stories. Then, if you have gained her attention, touch delicately on any concerns you have. If you want to ask the caseworker to do something for you or your foster child, try to make it a reasonable request.

Do not complain to the caseworker about "the system." She is just as frustrated as you are and neither of you can make changes. Use the local foster parent association as a resource if you want to change the system.

One foster parent said, "Respect is a two-way street. If you treat the case-worker or social worker with respect, you will get treated in a more respect-ful way." When talking to the caseworker, find good things to say about your foster child and about the biological family. This optimistic view will be helpful in your relationship with the caseworker and it will bring posi-tive attention to the foster child.

KEEPING IN TOUCH

> I've known this child and her two brothers for eight months. I just want to know how she's doing after she leaves me. I hope she gets a good teacher and her art talents are encouraged. She's such a cute little kid. I want her to do well.

Many foster parents retain a great interest in their foster children after they leave. They frequently take them to events, attend school concerts and graduations, and even help raise the child's own children. "I took her and the baby to the appointment, because I knew if I didn't, nobody else would," said a former foster father.

The biological family and foster family often become friends. Young bio-logical mothers may seem like children themselves. "With my last little one, her mother wanted me to adopt the baby and herself. I told her I couldn't do that, but I've always liked her a lot. I still see them about once a month." Many foster families make sure that former foster children have happy holidays and birthdays. They may have an annual summer picnic and in-vite whole families.

If you are afraid that your foster child will not be safe after returning home, and you want to be available for emergencies, talk about it while the child is with you. It may or may not be appropriate. You should let the case-worker know about your plans.

SENDING BACK HOME

> I know I don't have anything to say about it, but I really don't think she should be sent back to that mother. The house is dirty and noisy. The school is terrible. I think that she's scared to go back. I wish I could talk to the judge.

Look again at your motivation for being a foster parent. Did you want to give this child a safe home for a few months and help her reunite with the biological family? If so, did you talk positively about the family and say nice things to the mother on the phone? Or did you learn to love the child so much that you want to keep her, to raise her your own way, to have her company and see her smiling face every day?

Try to straighten out your own motivations and be realistic about this child's biological home. If you still feel that it is unsafe, talk to the caseworker. In some cases, foster parents may be allowed to speak to the judge.

Your concern may be due partly to worrying about how you, yourself, will feel if she leaves. That is called "separation anxiety" and it is quite natural. You can get helpful advice about your own anxieties by talking to experienced foster parents. Experienced foster parents get used to children coming and going. They seldom have much concern about separation, or about the child going back home.

GETTING ANGRY

> Sometimes I get really angry with this kid. She's so stubborn. I guess she knows how to get me going. I have to try all the methods I can think of to keep from shouting at her. Sometimes I'm afraid I'm going to hit her.

Foster parents get angry, just like everyone else. The important thing is how you manage that anger. Think back to the last time that you got angry with this child. Did you count to ten? Did you take a few deep breaths? If not, would that have helped? You can use the same techniques you teach the children for handling your own anger. Think of the consequences of shouting, of insulting the child, or of hitting the child. Are the consequences worth the moment of satisfaction?

If you have been angry, either at the child or in the child's presence, wait until you cool off to talk about it. Then do talk to the child about it. If you lost your temper, tell the child you are sorry and explain why. If you kept your temper, tell the child how difficult that was and what you did to control yourself.

If you get so angry that you become abusive, you run the risk of losing the foster child and also losing your certification as a foster parent. If you feel that is likely to happen in the near future, talk to the caseworker. Perhaps the caseworker will be able to arrange a formal or an informal respite, allowing the child to be away from you on a regular schedule. Possibly the child should be moved to another foster home.

NOT GETTING DISCOURAGED

> I've had three different foster children. One went into a different foster home and one went home to her mother. It doesn't seem like I helped those two kids. And I get real discouraged about the one I've got now.

One thing to do if you are feeling discouraged is to try to change your thought processes. You got into foster parenting in order to give kids a period to mature and change for the better. It is hard to measure success with children. The child may have gained a lot from the time in your home, yet how would you know? Did you get his cavities filled, his school-work caught up? Did you help him stop wetting the bed? These sorts of accomplishments are hard to measure. Try to find ways to measure small successes.

Most children do not realize that they have had a good experience in foster care. They may feel that they were being punished. Many children are focused on going back to their original home. When they leave, they may look very happy about going back home. Do not expect children to say or show their appreciation.

CASEWORKERS—DO THEY KNOW WHAT THEY'RE DOING?

My sister and I are both foster mothers and we have the same caseworker. She always seems totally confused. What are the qualifications to be a caseworker?

Some foster parents are disappointed in their caseworkers, and some foster parents have enormous praise for them. Everyone agrees that the job of a caseworker is difficult. Children are usually unhappy and biological families are usually difficult. Your agency may use a different title, but the caseworkers usually have a college degree and some experience in the field. Many caseworkers feel that the pay is too low and their caseloads are too large.

The caseworker's job is not scientific. A caseworker evaluates a family and decides, usually on the spot, if a child can stay in that home or not. There is no test to give the family in order to determine their degree of neglect or abuse. There is no scale for disturbance regarding unsupervised adolescents. The caseworker makes a decision and the judge usually accepts that decision. So caseworkers have a lot of responsibility.

Some foster parents advise that you try to make friends with the caseworker, instead of loading more criticism on her. Assume that most of the problems you are having are not the caseworker's fault. Thank her for her efforts.

ALLEGATIONS OF ABUSE

I thought we were doing pretty well. Candy was in fourth grade. She had friends and she went on trips with us. Then she told her caseworker that my husband was touching her. She was taken out of the home that day, and we've been in court seven times since then.

If a foster child feels he or she is being abused and reports that to the caseworker, that is called an "allegation." In other words, the child has accused the foster family of abuse. It is possible that the child is actually being abused. It appears that this does occur, from time to time. Foster families may have the same kind of stresses that were present in the biological home.

A second possibility is that some activities, such as hugging and kissing, were misinterpreted. Foster children who were formerly sexually abused are likely to misinterpret your actions as sexual in nature. The third possibility is that the child has become angry at the foster parents and has accused them of abuse maliciously. Such a foster child may know that the allegation will result in excitement and attention.

Usually when there has been an allegation, the legal system will remove the child and there will be an investigation. If there is evidence that abuse has occurred, the abuser will be charged and there will be a trial. Foster parents agree that allegations are heart wrenching. It is a terrible thing for a family to go through. There are lawyers who may be helpful and there are support groups. Your local foster parent association can advise.

It is important to avoid allegations if possible. Make sure that no one in your home is actually abusing your foster child. Make sure that there is no hugging and kissing of children over the age of five. Make sure that you do not ever hit a child in an attempt at discipline. Watch carefully when another person joins your household to be sure that some form of mistreatment does not start.

AGING OUT

My own kids lived at home, off and on, until they were about twenty-six or twenty-seven. They needed help buying a car, paying rent, and balancing a checkbook. Who's going to do that with this kid?

In most states, foster care ends at the age of eighteen. It may end before if the child runs away or drifts back to the biological family. The government does not want to keep foster children in care until they are in their mid-twenties, and the children would not want to stay. In order to smooth the transition to independence, states are beginning to develop after-care programs. In some communities there are special apartments for these youngsters, where they can receive some attention from a professional for several years.

If you have an older teenage foster child, you can help plan for the future. It may be appropriate to transfer the child from a regular high school into an occupational school where a trade can be learned. A child who learns to be a dental technician or a practical nurse will always be able to earn a living.

If the child were to remain in your home after "aging out," there might be special funding while the child is in full-time school. After that, in most cases, you would need to arrange with the child to pay rent. You can be an enormous help, as a child becomes independent, in helping him or her to get health insurance, job applications, and other paperwork completed.

FUTURE OF FOSTER CARE

Sometimes I really wonder what's going to happen to all these kids. Most of my women friends work full time and they could never do what I've done with foster children.

The number of children in foster care in this country has been increasing. However, most child care experts now agree that children should be kept with their own families whenever possible. Preventive programs, which help at-risk families to learn about raising children, are quite helpful. Unfortunately, they are not yet widely available. Studies have shown that preventive programs decrease the number of children in foster care.

When problems do begin to occur in a family, efforts are now made to strengthen the original family before a child is removed from the home. Psychological and social work services are provided. These programs also may help adults get a job and get off drugs. When a child enters foster care, agencies and judges are developing new approaches to treatment, so that improvement will occur more quickly and the child can return home. If a child cannot return home, a permanent plan needs to be developed.

The most optimistic view for the next century is that fewer children would need to be removed from their homes. Preventive programs would allow more children to live in loving, nurturing homes with their biological families. For those who are removed, a short period of directed care and quick movement through the court system would allow reunification or permanent planning within a short time frame.

WHAT DO OUTCOME STUDIES SHOW?

My wife says J.R.'s going to be in jail when he grows up, but I think maybe that he'll be all right. Sometimes he does drive us crazy. His parents sure messed him up. Do a lot of these kids end up in jail? Is there anything we can do to make sure that he doesn't?

There are no studies to tell us exactly what happens to children who have been in foster care. Unfortunately, some former foster children do end up in jail, yet many others go back home and never have any more problems. There are studies going on now that should help answer this question in the future. Large studies can show what happens to the children and what approaches work best.

Most child care professionals estimate that about half of today's foster children will end up earning a living and living in a family. Of the rest, some will end up on welfare and ten to fifteen percent will be either homeless or in jail.

There are some approaches to foster care that seem to show good results. Children seem to do best if they are kept in foster care less than a year. During that time the child can get help with physical health, mental health, and education. The child will be a year older and better able to do well at home and at school when discharged from foster care.

TIPS FROM OTHER FOSTER PARENTS

> I don't know any other foster parents and most of my friends think I'm nuts to be doing this. Sometimes I just want to ask other foster parents how to do things. I love this kid so much and I get so frustrated.

One place to turn for advice is foster parent associations in your own community. There is also a national organization, the National Foster Parent Association, with a newsletter. The Internet has many sites where foster parents ask questions and other foster parents answer. Here are some tips from various foster parents.

Teach self-control, don't impose control.

In conversation, respond to the child, not to your own agenda.

Don't ask yes or no questions; ask, "What good thing happened today?"

Show the child you care what he or she thinks.

Model good listening skills, it helps children learn to listen.

Let the child explore as much as you can.

Do not act superior. Do not say, "You're too young." Respect the child's opinions.

Do not use negative assumptions like, "You always. . . . "

Help the child learn to dress and feed himself or herself.

Avoid doing anything for the child that he or she is capable of doing.

Be proud of the child's accomplishments.

Teach a good healthy self-concept.

Just love them.

Take at least one picture per year of every foster child and store them with the child's records.

SAFETY

> I worry more about these kids than I ever did about my own kids. I'm so afraid that a foster child will get hit by a car and it will look like my fault. And I know it will really feel like my fault, if anything happens.

Good foster parents are always concerned about safety. For one thing, the age of their children may change abruptly. Safety issues for a toddler are quite different from safety issues for a teenager. Try to sit down and go over a list of safety concerns every so often. All parents have safety concerns, and all parents feel responsible when a child is injured. Foster parents need to be especially careful, because the children may be unpredictable.

Also, foster children are often not good at following rules. After advising a child about safe behavior, you will need to make sure the child follows through. Whether or not a foster child is being malicious, he or she will be unlikely to follow all your rules without some monitoring on your part. In addition, foster children are often hyperactive or obsessive. These conditions, and others, affect a person's judgment. Such a child may dash into the street with little concern about oncoming traffic.

If you go to the emergency room with an injured foster child, be prepared for some questions about the way you are raising this child. Try not to let your feelings be hurt. Emergency room doctors need to think first about the safety of the children they are seeing.

MAKING A CHILD RESILIENT

Diego has the potential to get through life and be a real success. His family, though, is something else. It's possible they'll just drag him down. I want to help him become so tough and so smart that, when he goes back home, he'll still do well.

Children are known to be more resilient if they do well in school, care about others, have ties with at least one adult, and have an optimistic outlook. Anything you can do to create or strengthen these personality traits in your foster child will be helpful. Probably the day-to-day influence of good foster parents is more important than therapy, school, home visits, and other activities for foster children.

Studies do indicate that success for a former foster child may be mixed with some persistent problems. Marriages may fail and family relationships may be strained. An adult who has grown up in foster care may complain of nightmares or of great sadness, such as victims of a war might feel.

GRIEVING

Oh, Carlos left last week. What am I going to do? He's been a part of our life for two and a half years. I don't know if I can stand it. I can't sleep at night. I'm so angry and confused.

Even though the nature of foster care is that children come and go, it may be quite disturbing when a child leaves. You probably know, in a logical way, that Carlos will be all right. You have probably already checked with his new foster mother and she is getting along fine with him.

Most likely the first emotion you had, when you heard he was going, was anger. It is easy to be angry, as a foster parent. You might be angry at the biological parents, the judge, the caseworker, or the system. You are grieving for this foster child. You loved him and now he is gone. After a loss, people go through a roller-coaster ride of emotions. One moment they are angry, the next moment they are praying to have the child back. Every time another adult is willing to listen, you tell that person how awful you feel and how frustrated you are.

At some point, no matter how sad and confused you have been, you will begin to resolve some things in your mind. You will tell yourself that Carlos is gone and that your life will go on. If you are staying in the foster care business, your mood will improve the minute a caseworker calls and asks, "Do you have a minute?" If you have had a chance to grieve, you will move on, accept a new foster child, and learn to love that child.

17

Particular Concerns
of Foster Children

Foster children have many concerns, and sometimes it appears that no one listens to these concerns. Most foster children worry about their status in the community. Most are impoverished and behind in their education; also, their behavior is often immature.

Foster children do not know where they belong. They feel that their own families do not love them. No one else seems to love them. They also worry about the future. Try to anticipate questions that a foster child may have. Be ready to listen, whenever the child feels like asking you questions. If you cannot help, try to find out who can help.

GETTING ADVICE

Right now I need advice on how to get a part-time job. Last year I wanted to know how to get some new clothes. I don't like my caseworker and my foster parents don't seem to take the time. Sometimes I just want to talk things over and try to figure out what my future will be. Who can I talk to?

Lots of kids, when they get fed up with their parents or foster parents, turn to their friends for advice. You have to be careful about doing that, because they may give you bad advice. Still, talking things over with other young people can be helpful, as long as you remember that you do not need to follow their advice.

There may be ways to encourage your foster parents to help. Consider going to one of them and asking to set an appointment to sit down and talk. Tell them you have a lot of things on your mind and you just want them to listen and help you come up with answers. You might be surprised that your foster mom or dad would be flattered if you asked for advice.

Other adults might help, if you asked them. Try asking your biological grandmother or your foster parents' next-door neighbor to help you work some things out. They might be honored to do that. So, the first step is to find an adult you respect and set a time to sit down with that person.

When you meet, start out with some neutral topic that will get the person's attention, like baseball or sewing. Then tell the person your general areas of concern. That might be education, career plans, health, sex, or other things. Try to keep the discussion practical and short. An adult may offer advice, but the best help will be if the adult encourages you to find solutions for yourself.

If the meeting was helpful, thank the person. Ask if you can meet again in a few weeks. Say that you are still thinking a lot of things over and that you feel better having talked to someone. On the other hand, you may be disappointed in such a conversation. Some adults are quick to tell you what you should do and will not listen to your thoughts and doubts. Thank that person anyway. He or she has probably tried to help.

If you do identify someone who can advise you and help you, consider asking to meet on a regular basis. Being able to form a relationship like this is very important for your future.

STAYING OUT OF TROUBLE

I've been hanging around with some kids. They're a lot of fun, but they don't have any rules. They do some shoplifting and they drink a lot of alcohol. I really like to be with them, but I'm afraid I'm going to get into trouble.

Friends are very important. You probably do not want to throw away the friends you have. Your challenge is to keep your involvement with these friends and still stay out of trouble. One suggestion is to get a wider circle of friends. Try to find some different kids to spend a little time with. Join a club or go to the local community center and sign up for activities. Sports and other physical activities are excellent ways to meet people and to stay out of trouble. Young people who practice a sport tend to be law abiding.

If there are after-school programs for little kids, see if you can volunteer to help in one of those programs. Young people who are good volunteers are often offered paying jobs, so this volunteer project of yours may turn into a summer job.

If you are thinking of dropping out of school, think again. Kids who drop out of school before they graduate almost always end up in trouble. You might, however, think about changing from an academic program to an occupational program.

If you are involved with friends who are shoplifting and drinking alcohol, you need to resist doing these things yourself. Foster children often have problems if they go to court. The judge probably already knows you, and if the judge thinks you are starting to get into trouble your placement may be changed.

HOW OTHER KIDS REACT TO FOSTER CHILDREN

I always feel like everyone knows my business. Everybody knows that the person who picks me up at school is my caseworker. Everyone knows that my biological parents are in trouble a lot. What can I do to feel better about myself?

Getting through the teenage years can be difficult for everyone. Lots of teens feel uncomfortable from time to time. You might find that people are paying less attention to you and your activities than you think. Perhaps you can think of some changes that would make you feel better, such as having the caseworker pick you up at home.

Also, lots of kids who are not in foster care have lousy families. They may be embarrassed that their families drive old cars, or they may be embarassed that their parents yell at each other and drink too much.

Do you have a plan for the next few years? Are you going to get your high school degree, go to junior college, and get a job? Is your caseworker helping you to fulfill these plans? If so, you should feel a lot of pride that you are moving towards your goal of independence. And you are succeeding, even without the help of your biological parents. Take pride in your accomplishments and focus on your future.

ABUSE IN FOSTER HOMES

What do I do if I feel like I'm being abused? My foster dad never really hits me, but he yells at me and makes fun of me? It's gotten worse since he lost his job. I feel like I used to feel when I was with my own dad.

Abuse does occur in foster homes. Foster children often hate to report the foster family, because they will have to move somewhere else. If you are really being physically abused, like being beaten, slapped, or kicked, you should tell your caseworker. That sort of thing tends to get worse, and if you do not get hurt, someone else will.

If it is still at the yelling stage, talk to your foster mom about it. Tell her how you are feeling and ask if there is anything you can say or do that will help. She may have some suggestions like keeping the rock music turned down or keeping the kitchen cleaned up. Then try talking to your foster dad. Tell him the steps you have already taken and ask him to try to treat you better in the future.

Are there other places for you to spend some of your time while your foster dad is upset? How about going to the public library or the neighborhood center? Would this be a good time to get a part-time job, which you have been thinking about?

If your foster father was good to you in the past, remember the good times. Suggest to him that you and he could go to a game together or go for a bike ride. Then, when he does get upset, try to go outside while he is yelling. Even though you feel like none of this is your fault, it is worth trying to get along with him if you can.

SEXUAL FEELINGS IN THE FOSTER HOME

> I think I'm in love with someone in my foster family. I can't think about anyone else. I can't sleep at night. It's a great feeling, but it's scary.

It is very common for sexual feeling to develop between people who live in the same home. As these are not your own relatives, it may feel quite natural. Perhaps you just have a "crush" on that other person. This can happen to you whether you are eight years old or eighteen. It can happen if the person is male or female. Try not to do anything that you will regret later. Think things over carefully and then try to get over these feelings. Get out of the house as much as you can. Spend time with your friends or get active in sports.

Another possibility is that this member of the foster family has said that he or she is in love with you. Now both of you have to consider carefully whether a relationship is appropriate. A romantic relationship with someone much older is usually not appropriate. In fact, it may not be legal. Talk it over with the person and then talk it over with the caseworker. Sexual relationships can always be delayed. Do not let anyone pressure you into having sex.

The third possibility is that a foster mother or foster father wants to have sex with you. This can be dangerous. If they want you to have sex with them, say no and call the caseworker. If you want to have sex with them, do not do it. If it is a foster brother or sister or another young adult in the home, you must talk it over with the caseworker.

GAINING WEIGHT

> When I was a little kid I was kind of skinny. Now I feel like I'm huge. I eat all the time, too. Soda, candy, chips, and pizza are everywhere. And I can't stop eating them.

During the teenage years many people gain weight. Some weight gain is normal, because as you grow up you naturally gain weight. However, if an adult is overweight, that problem probably started in the teenage years. So excessive weight gain is something teenagers should watch out for.

Sometimes foster children take medication that causes weight gain. Some medication used to control behavior, such as antidepressants, can affect the appetite. The medication may be quite helpful, so the weight gain may be a small price to pay. Birth control pills and birth control shots can also cause weight gain. Good eating habits can usually prevent weight gain.

The best way to keep your weight down or to lose weight is to eat less and exercise more. Exercise, by itself, does not take weight off. It seems that a diet that contains five servings of fruits and vegetables a day helps keep a person from over-eating. In other words, if you fill up on carrots and apples, you will not be so hungry for pizza.

There are some ways to lose weight that you should avoid. That includes making yourself vomit, using laxatives, and smoking cigarettes. None of those are healthy ways to lose weight. And remember, not everyone is a super-skinny model type.

THINKING BACK OVER LIFE

I've been treated really bad all my life. My mom yelled at me, my dad used to beat me, my uncles had sex with me. Will I ever turn out normal?

The first thing to remember is that those things that happened were not your fault. People tend to blame the victim and that's not right. So if you were treated badly, it was their fault. And if they got into trouble when someone found out, that was not your fault, either.

You may be getting a lot of help already. Counseling is usually part of the job of the caseworker. Foster parents are often really good at letting you talk about your past. One thing to try is to sit down with people like that and see if they can help you.

On the other hand, you may have already decided that these people cannot help. They may not be very understanding. They may not be able to keep secrets. See if your agency has a program to find a special adult to meet with you. This may be a mentor, a big sister or brother, or a friendship person. If you start getting together with someone, take a little time to get to know that person. Then ask if he or she could help you.

If you do not have a social worker or a professional counselor, ask for one. Tell your caseworker that you have a lot of stuff that you want to talk about. Usually counseling is available for foster children, but it may take a little time to work this out.

GETTING AHEAD IN LIFE

I want to be a big success as an adult. I want fancy clothes, a good marriage, a nice house, and a good job. What will help me do well as an adult?

Some former foster children have ended up being quite successful. Here are some suggestions that might help you.

The first thing to do is postpone having children. That applies to both boys and girls. Having a baby is a big responsibility. It brings the rest of your plans to a halt. You have to stop moving ahead and start raising a child. Always use condoms if you are having sex.

Look for a mentor. A mentor is an adult who can help you with your life. A mentor is someone you can talk with who will be understanding and helpful. This person may be your foster mother's sister or it may your boss in a fast-food restaurant. If you treat that person with respect, he or she will respect you and will be happy to help you out.

Make an appointment at a clinic for medical care and family planning. As you grow up, you need to begin to make your own medical appointments and then get to the clinic on time. You probably can continue to go to the same clinic you used in foster care after you leave care. Have your foster parents help you with this planning when you are getting ready to leave.

Get mental health care if you need it. Did you take pills for hyperactivity as a little child? Perhaps you still need medicine to slow you down. Are you depressed? Maybe you need medicine for that. Go to a regular clinic and tell people there how you feel. They will arrange for counseling or mental health clinic visits. Do not think there is something wrong with you because you are on medication. Lots of people take medication and live terrific lives.

Get all the education you can. Everyone benefits from education. You learn to write, to get organized, to think in a logical way, and to talk clearly. Go to a local junior college after you finish high school. Take a few classes or become a full-time student. If you cannot continue with school, postpone it briefly, then start again whenever you can.

Certain attitudes are important for people, as they grow up. It is important to care about others and indicate that you care about them. This is called "prosocial behavior" and it is similar to the golden rule. Act toward others the way you want them to act toward you. It really works.

AFTER FOSTER CARE

What's going to happen when I turn eighteen? I'm excited about growing up, but I don't have any plans yet. My foster mom says I haven't got much common sense.

In most cases foster care ends at age eighteen. That is good and bad, as far as foster children are concerned. It is nice to be old enough to make decisions, but it can be hard to figure out what to do. While you are a teenager, try to learn the things you will need. Here are some ideas.

Learn about balancing a checkbook, paying bills, opening a bank account, and keeping information for taxes. When you are old enough, ask your foster parents to tell you how they do things and ask them to help you get started.

When you are able to save money for purchases, in your late teenage years, be careful what you buy. Buy a small television set. Buy some work clothes and some clothes to relax in. Try to stock up on underwear and socks.

Learn how to cook simple meals. Ask your foster mother to recommend a cookbook that is practical and easy to understand, and use it to practice making basic meals. Have your foster mother help you learn to understand labels on food and to understand what makes for a nutritious diet.

Unless you expect to have a car and a driver's license, get information about public transportation. Learn about neighborhoods where you could live and reasonable rental costs for rooms or apartments.

Talk to the caseworker about programs that will be helpful to you. Can a caseworker maintain some contact for a few years? This will be good for you, if that can be arranged. Is there an apartment complex where other former foster children live and where they get some help? Can you find a roommate to share the expenses and to keep you company?

Your present foster family may be willing to continue to advise you and to keep an eye on your health and your finances with you. There are some states that allow you to stay in foster care until you are a little older if you continue to go to school.

If you want help from people your own age, see if there is a support group for older foster children. Also, get on the Internet and read, as foster children talk about their problems and offer each other solutions. Remember that, on the Internet, you do not know the qualifications of the person who is advising you. So be careful about taking advice too seriously.

BIOLOGICAL FAMILY

I love my Mom and I do want to keep in touch with her. Sometimes when I see her, I get so upset about the younger kids and their problems that I can't sleep at night. My stepfather used to hit me a lot, and now I think he hits the younger kids. What should I do?

Loving your biological family is appropriate. These people will always be family to you. As you get older, you may be able to help them to cope. Right now, your best bet is to keep yourself going, learn to cope with your own life, and try to have short visits with your biological family.

Do you dream about getting older, buying a home, and letting your biological brother and sisters move in? That is a reasonable dream, but now is the time to try to get your own life together. Meanwhile, try to see your biological family on holidays and plan regular short visits. Remember to send birthday cards. Pay special attention to younger brothers and sisters and try to go to their school activities when you can.

Try very hard not to drift back to living with your biological family. That is a step backward for most foster children who have grown up in foster care. Let the caseworker advise you about that. If the caseworker says not to go back home, then follow that advice.

PREGNANCY

I'm pregnant. It's so neat to be having a baby. I'm taking vitamins and going to the clinic. But I don't know what's going to happen after the baby comes. My boyfriend wants us to live together, but I'm only sixteen. My foster mother wants me to stay with her. I'm afraid someone will take my baby away.

First, most adults would say you are not ready to have a baby. It will be very hard to get your own life together and also raise a child. However, it appears that you are committed to having the baby. It is important to take vitamins and do everything else the doctor recommends. Do not smoke, drink alcohol, or take drugs. You do want this child to get off to the best possible start.

Basically the law says that every parent and every child have the right to live together. You should not sign any papers that take away your rights to the child. Do not sign a voluntary placement agreement even if the caseworker tells you to. Signing that will take away your control over the child.

If you are happy in your foster home, that is probably the best place to start raising the child. Your boyfriend will be around to help, but so will your foster family. When you turn eighteen, you may be ready to move out of foster care.

Make plans now to start using birth control as soon as the baby is born. If you are not careful, there will be another baby. Talk to the clinic about your concern and then remember to take action as soon as the baby comes.

Over the next few months, learn as much as you can about raising children. Go to parenting classes and make your boyfriend go with you. Go to the library and find books about children. Read everything you can and talk to everyone you know. Good luck.

COLLEGE

All my friends are going to college. What about me?

In most cases, you cannot start college until you graduate from high school. Occasionally, a high school student can take college courses and that is usually free. If you have dropped out of high school but want to start college, see about getting a high school equivalency degree. You will need to do some studying before taking the exam. Go to your local high school to get information on this.

Junior colleges often have students who have grown up without much money. Talk to the admissions department and see if you can afford to go there. You will need to work part time to earn some money. You may also qualify for welfare, in some form, or for medical benefits. Local junior colleges offer very practical courses. You can take a nursing program or a welding program or a criminal justice program. Then when you graduate, you will have a good chance of getting a steady job.

If you feel that you could do well in a four-year college and you have gotten good grades in high school, you might qualify for a full scholarship plus loans. If your grades in high school were not so great, enter a junior college or a community college. If you work hard and get good grades there, you will be able to transfer to a four-year college.

RUNNING AWAY

One of my friends, who used to be in a foster home, ran away. Now he's homeless. Sometimes he stays here, with my foster family. He doesn't go to school. I'm not sure if he's very happy.

Some foster children end up homeless as they get older. How does a homeless person survive? Such a person may work a little to earn some money, may beg for money, or may steal. If a homeless person finds a warm bed or a meal, it will probably be in a shelter.

Homeless young people may feel quite free, but they are very unsafe. Someone may steal their possessions, rape them, or beat them up. Many homeless persons end up stealing in order to survive and then get arrested. Studies show that homelessness leads to crime, and crime leads to jail.

A homeless person probably cannot get any health care and will not be able to get prescriptions filled. The person will not be able to have a steady relationship with another person. The homeless person will not be able to keep or care for a pet. There will be many cold and sleepless nights.

So what should a foster teen who is about to drift into homelessness do? Try to find ways to change your life for the better. Should you be living in a group home? Should you be in a vocational school? Go outside and get lots of exercise. Do not sit in your room watching television.

If a young person is already homeless, there are groups that can help. Call the local number for runaway and homeless youth. Get reconnected with adults and see if you can put your life back on track.

SUICIDE

Life has been rotten lately. I'm miserable. I'm mad at everybody. I might kill myself. That would sure get back at them.

The first thing to tell you is, "Do not do it." Suicide is a terrible thing. Death is final. Even if your life seems drab and uninteresting now, things can always get better. Remember that whoever loves you will feel bad if you die. So, instead of killing yourself, go to someone who loves you and tell that person what you are thinking about and why. Figure out a way to stay alive for a few more months.

If you are unhappy because of splitting up with a girlfriend or boyfriend, remember that there will be others as you grow older. You will look back on this person and wonder why it upset you so much to split up.

If you are unhappy because you think you might be gay, try to get some information. Many gay men and women have great normal lives. Try to connect with someone who is gay, so you can find out what it is really like. Many people are uncomfortable about homosexuality, so if the first person you talk to turns you away, try another person. Eventually, you will find a person who can listen to your problems and advise you or comfort you.

If school is going badly, try not to feel like it is your fault. You have done well just to get this far in life. You have a lot of strength and a lot of talent. Many adults who did not finish school or finished school a little later in life are quite happy and successful.

Are you worried because you are leaving foster care? There are many services out there for persons like you, but you may really have to search them out. Can you get a free college education? Yes, that is available, but not easy to find. Can you get on welfare and find an apartment? Probably you can. Can you get a job? There is a job out there for everyone.

If there are weapons in the house, ask your foster parents to remove them or lock them away, so that you will not be tempted to use them. If you can sit down and talk to your foster parents about your feelings, of course that is what you should do. If you really cannot talk to them, try to find another adult who will give you some comfort. Go to a medical clinic, a family planning clinic, a mental health clinic, or even to a police station. Tell people there your problem and ask for help.

NOT GETTING RESPECT BY THE JUDGE

I have been to court every year since I was eight. The judge never talks to me or asks me what I think. I don't think that's fair.

One common area of concern for foster children is that they are not allowed to decide what they want to do. When they go to court, the social worker and probation officer talk to the judge and the judge makes a decision. Many foster children want to have some control of their own future.

It is a fact that the judge is not required to ask you whether you want to stay in foster care, go to a group home, or go back to your parents. The law says that persons under the age of eighteen are not old enough to make that kind of decision. Obviously, that is pretty frustrating if you have a reasonable plan.

If you feel like you want to make a change or if you want to stay where you are, try to talk to the caseworker or the probation officer alone. Plan what you are going to say. Use a mature voice and speak slowly and clearly. If you convince these professionals, they will convince the judge.

FOSTER CHILDREN WHO HAVE DONE WELL

I've known a lot of foster children and most of them have not turned out very well. One friend is in jail and another is homeless. What will happen to me?

Probably some of the kids you've known are doing fine now. They have gone to college and gotten married. You may not hear much good news like that, yet it does happen.

One former foster child said, "I've been in gangs and I've been in jail. I've taken drugs. But then one day I said I should pull myself together. I decided I had gained a lot of experience and now it was time to settle down." This person discovered some inner strength and used that strength in good ways.

You need to plan your life. Get all the education you can get. Education has a mysterious effect of making young people grow up. Find persons who love you and ask for their help. Spend less time watching television and more time reading. Get some physical activity every day.

HELPING OTHER FOSTER CHILDREN

I'm getting my life together. I've started to think that I can help other kids like me. Are there groups out there for foster kids?

Some communities have support groups for foster children or for former foster children. There are many sites on the Internet where foster children write and ask for help. If you do answer these children, try to be encouraging. In most cases, children benefit most by trying to tolerate the situation they are in, rather than trying to change it.

If you are no longer a foster child, but used to be one, consider becoming a mentor or a big brother or big sister for a foster child. If you have a home and you are earning a living, consider becoming a foster parent. It is very likely that you have a lot of wisdom and can help other children who have been removed from their homes.

ADVICE FROM FOSTER CHILDREN AND FORMER FOSTER CHILDREN

Many foster children have advice for foster parents, for other foster children, for professionals, or for the general public. This is a list of suggestions taken from conversations with foster children or former foster children.

Treat foster children with respect. If you don't give respect, I don't give it back.
Don't expect me to be real quiet. I need to make a lot of noise.
Don't give me lectures.
When you ask a question, give me time to think of the answer.
Shoot baskets with me or play catch with me.
Don't say bad things about my mother.
I don't like it when you yell at me.
I like to stay up late.
Don't be so strict.
Help me learn to control my anger.
Help me get ready for the future.

Resources

Albrecht, Donna. *Raising a Child Who Has a Physical Disability*. New York: John Wiley and Sons, 1995.

Appelstein, Charles. *The Gus Chronicles*. Needham, MA: Albert E. Trieschman Center, 1994.

Clark, Lynn. *SOS Help for Parents*. Bowling Green, OH: Parents Press, 1996.

Davies, Nancy Millichap. *Foster Care*. New York: Franklin Watts, 1994.

Falke, Joseph. *Living in a Foster Home*. New York: Rosen Publishing, 1995.

Fuller, Cheri. *Helping Your Child Succeed in Public School*. Colorado Springs: Focus on the Family, 1993.

Glenn, Stephen, and Michael Brock. *Seven Strategies for Developing Capable Students*. Rocklin, CA: Prima, 1998.

Grossman, Elmer. *Everyday Pediatrics for Parents*. Berkeley: Celestial Arts, 1996.

Hallowell, Edward. *When You Worry about the Child You Love*. New York: Simon and Schuster, 1996.

Joseph, Joanne. *The Resilient Child*. New York: Plenum Press, 1994.

Joslin, Karen Renshaw, and Mary Bunting Decher. *Positive Parenting Your Teens*. New York: Fawcett Columbine, 1997.

Kaye, Kenneth. *Family Rules*. New York: St. Martin's Press, 1984.

LaVert, Suzanne. *When Your Child Has a Chronic Illness*. New York: Bantam Doubleday Dell, 1995.

Levine, Katherine Gordy. *When Good Kids Do Bad Things*. New York: Pocket Books, 1991.

Paul, Henry. *When Kids Are Mad, Not Bad*. New York: Berkley Books, 1995.

Pelzer, Dave. *A Child Called "It."* Deerfield Beach, FL: Health Communications, 1995.

Pelzer, Dave. *A Foster Child's Search for the Love of a Family*. Deerfield Beach, FL: Health Communications, 1997.

Regoli, Robert M., and John D. Hewitt. *Delinquency in Society—A Child Centered Approach*. New York: McGraw-Hill, 1991.

Riley, Douglas. *The Defiant Child*. Dallas: Taylor Publishing, 1997.

Schiff, Donald, and Steven Shelov. *American Academy of Pediatrics—Guide to Your Child's Symptoms*. New York: Villard, 1997.

Schor, D. *American Academy of Pediatrics—Caring for Your School-Age Child*. New York: Bantam, 1995.

Shelov, Steven. *American Academy of Pediatrics—Caring for Your Baby and Young Child*. New York: Bantam, 1998.

Turecki, Stanley. *The Difficult Child*. New York: Bantam Books, 1989.

Weitzman, Elizabeth. *Let's Talk about Foster Homes*. New York: Rosen Publishing, 1996.

Zigelman, David. *The Pocket Pediatrician*. New York: Doubleday, 1995.

ORGANIZATIONS

Child Welfare League of America
440 First St. NW, Third Floor
Washington, DC 20001–2085

National Foster Parents Association
Karen Jorgenson
P.O. Box 81
Alpha, OH 45301

Index

About the Author

SUSAN McNAIR BLATT, M.D., is the Medical Director of the House of Good Shepherd in Utica, New York, a child welfare agency, and is an Adjunct Professor at Utica College.